D0987064

Praise for *The End of Trauma*

"Everything you know about trauma—about how human beings deal with the worst things that can possibly happen to them—is probably wrong. One book can fix that, and this is the one. The world's expert on human resilience has written a powerful, important, and fascinating book that explains how ordinary people take arms against a sea of troubles, and by opposing, end them."

—Daniel Gilbert,
New York Times–bestselling author,
Stumbling on Happiness

"George Bonanno has hit a home run. With a blend of page-turning stories, illuminating examples, and cutting-edge science, *The End of Trauma* is guaranteed to change your mind about the sources and prevalence of trauma. Reading this gorgeously written book will make you appreciate your own mind's flexibility and how to capitalize on it to become a more resilient person."

—Sonja Lyubomirsky, distinguished professor of
psychology, University of California, Riverside,
and author of *The How of Happiness*

"George Bonanno has done groundbreaking research on the psychology of resilience. In this book, he reveals how people can break free from the aftershocks of traumatic events. I can't think of a better time for his insights."

—Adam Grant,
#1 *New York Times*–bestselling author,
Think Again and *Option B*

"Bonanno is a master storyteller. *The End of Trauma* turns common sense on its head with impeccable science and a narrative like a suspense novel. If you or your loved ones have ever faced great adversity, this book is for you."

—Lisa Feldman Barrett,
author of *How Emotions Are Made*

"George Bonanno is a leading thinker about trauma and resilience. And in his new book *The End of Trauma*, he argues that much of what you think you know about trauma is wrong. Bonanno uses moving accounts of patients and his extensive knowledge of this field to make his case, offering an insight-filled new perspective on trauma, treatment, and resilience."

—Joseph LeDoux, author,
The Deep History of Ourselves

"George Bonanno is a rare scientist-researcher who knows how to systematically and deeply explore whatever he's attempting to understand while also being able to translate it into clear, easy-to-follow guidance. *The End of Trauma* was four decades in the making, and it was worth the wait."

—Patricia Watson,
National Center for PTSD

"*The End of Trauma* by George Bonanno is one of the most interesting, well-written, and clinically relevant books that I have read in recent years. It turns out that humans are far better at coping with traumatic events than we had thought. The book really soars when he tells the story of individuals who transcended terrible experiences and endured. A truly great book for everyone."

—Robert L. Leahy, director,
American Institute for Cognitive Therapy

"An instant classic in the science of PTSD. With keen insight, abundant sensitivity, and persuasive prose, Bonanno helps us understand why resilience isn't so much a trait as it is a process—one that requires flexibility and wisdom to manage effectively. By providing much of that wisdom, he helps open the door to resilience for everyone who has faced adversity and trauma."

—David DeSteno,
professor of psychology, Northeastern University

"In *The End of Trauma*, George Bonanno charts a brilliant and illuminating path forward in our understanding of trauma and how we find wisdom in resilience. This book will transform our understanding of the hardest times of life."

—Dacher Keltner,
professor of psychology, UC Berkeley

"A remarkable book. *The End of Trauma* deftly describes what George Bonanno and others have discovered about how people experience devastating experiences yet emerge psychologically unscathed. With the narrative drive of a gifted novelist, Bonanno tells the dramatic, inspiring stories of survivors of accidents, war, and terrorism who triumphed over trauma, and shows how the pragmatic, flexible application of certain emotion regulation skills can foster resilience."

—Richard J. McNally, professor of psychology
and director of clinical training, Harvard University

The End of Trauma

The End of Trauma

of

How the New Science of
Resilience Is Changing
How We Think About PTSD

GEORGE A. BONANNO

BASIC BOOKS

New York

Copyright © 2021 by George A. Bonanno
Cover design by Ann Kirchner
Cover images © seksan wangkeeree / Shutterstock.com; © Alexandru Nika / Shutterstock.com
Cover copyright © 2021 Hachette Book Group, Inc.

Hachette Book Group supports the right to free expression and the value of copyright. The purpose of copyright is to encourage writers and artists to produce the creative works that enrich our culture.

The scanning, uploading, and distribution of this book without permission is a theft of the author's intellectual property. If you would like permission to use material from the book (other than for review purposes), please contact permissions@hbgusa.com. Thank you for your support of the author's rights.

Basic Books
Hachette Book Group
1290 Avenue of the Americas, New York, NY 10104
www.basicbooks.com

Printed in the United States of America

First Edition: September 2021

Published by Basic Books, an imprint of Perseus Books, LLC, a subsidiary of Hachette Book Group, Inc. The Basic Books name and logo is a trademark of the Hachette Book Group.

The Hachette Speakers Bureau provides a wide range of authors for speaking events. To find out more, go to www.hachettespeakersbureau.com or call (866) 376-6591.

The publisher is not responsible for websites (or their content) that are not owned by the publisher.

Print book interior design by Jeff Williams

Library of Congress Cataloging-in-Publication Data

Names: Bonanno, George A., author.

Title: The end of trauma : how the new science of resilience is changing how we think about PTSD / George A. Bonanno.

Description: First edition. | New York : Basic Books, [2021] | Includes bibliographical references and index.

Identifiers: LCCN 2020057084 | ISBN 9781541674363 (hardcover) | ISBN 9781541674370 (ebook)

Subjects: LCSH: Post-traumatic stress disorder. | Psychic trauma. | Resilience (Personality trait).

Classification: LCC RC552.P67 B656 2021 | DDC 616.85/21—dc23

LC record available at https://lccn.loc.gov/2020057084

ISBNs: 978-1-5416-7436-3 (hardcover); 978-1-5416-7437-0 (ebook)

LSC-C

Printing 1, 2021

For Raphael and Angie

Contents

Contents

Author's Note

This book includes firsthand accounts of a number of courageous people who have endured extreme or potentially traumatic events. With the exception of Jed McGiffin and Maren Westphal, I have altered their names and personal details to preserve confidentiality.

Why Was I Doing Okay?

I first met Jed when he interviewed for the doctoral program in clinical psychology at Columbia University's Teachers College, where I'm a professor. Like most of the candidates I met that day, Jed was well dressed and respectful as he walked into my office. The fact that he *walked* into my office came as a bit of a surprise, though. I knew that Jed had been in a terrible accident that had almost killed him. I wasn't sure he was going to be *able* to walk.

Jed didn't say much about the accident that day. There were lots of other things to talk about. It wasn't until quite a while later that I learned the full story.

Five years earlier, Jed had been trying to make a living as a musician in New York. No small feat. As he put it, "I was a musician who was necessarily a waiter." Although he had been working at one of New York's finest restaurants, Babbo Ristorante in Greenwich Village, he was looking to make a change. He had just moved in with his girlfriend, Megan. She was studying nursing. Jed began to think about his longtime interest in psychology. He took a few classes at

City College uptown. It had gone well, and he planned to take a full load the next semester.

Thoughts about the future were circling around in Jed's mind as he completed a long shift on the night of December 21. The restaurant had just closed. It was around 1:30 a.m. Jed headed down to the basement to pick out some wine from the restaurant's sommelier as holiday gifts for his family. He found four nice bottles and stowed them away in his backpack before heading out the door.

The night was bitter cold. Jed pulled his hoodie snug and waited on the corner of West Eighth Street. The white light of the walk signal shimmered off the frozen pavement, and Jed made his way into the intersection. A garbage truck came around the corner, sudden and fast, and caught him. Before he knew it, he was down.

"I remember the whole thing, vividly," Jed told me. "I was knocked down by the front bumper and then pulled under by the front wheels. I went down kind of to the left, you know, my left leg went out, and I got run over by the front wheel."

The front wheel crushed Jed's leg. Then there was a brief pause.

One second.

Two seconds.

And then the truck's two double-axle rear wheels hit him.

"The whole twenty-five tons of truck . . . rolled over me."

Oddly, the four wine bottles in Jed's backpack remained intact. But Jed's leg and part of his hip were flattened into a mess of blood and bone. It was a brutal accident. He screamed wildly.

An emergency response team from the fire department was the first to arrive on the scene. They got there remarkably quickly, in a matter of just a few minutes.

Lieutenant Adrian Walsh found Jed and held his hand.

Jed remembers being acutely aware of the danger he was in.

"I knew it was life or death. I never passed out. I was screaming. I know I was screaming for a while."

Then he learned that the ambulance that would eventually take him to St. Vincent's Hospital was delayed. Although St. Vincent's was only six blocks away, the ambulance was locked up in traffic. The wait was excruciating.

"It was getting really scary. The fire department showed up and they shut down the whole thing. I very much remember the garbage truck. I could see from where I was lying that they'd stopped up the road, I could remember that really vividly."

Nothing much could be done until the ambulance arrived, but where was it?

"There was a lot of yelling. Lieutenant Walsh was yelling. She was trying to find a way to get me to the hospital. They were getting worried. She was yelling to the fire department. She was pointing to her vehicle, yelling, 'Can't we just put him in this thing, and take him to St. Vincent's?'"

With every minute that ticked by, Jed was in greater and greater danger. He had lost an enormous amount of blood. Lieutenant Walsh later speculated that if there was any luck at all on that fateful night, it was that Jed was lying on the icy cold pavement, which probably slowed the blood loss. Even so, Jed was bleeding profusely. The paramedics had to give him fifty units of blood, nearly five times the body's normal capacity.

It took twenty-five excruciating minutes for the ambulance to show up. For Jed, it was an eternity. He had no choice but to deal with it.

"I remember being sort of meditative on the pavement, like zoned in, maybe following my breath. I don't know what I was do-ing. I was in shock. There was a lot of furor going on. People were shouting, '*Put a rush on the bus!*' The bus is what they called the ambulance. There was this kind woman, Lieutenant Walsh, holding my hand, trying to keep me calm. And I was just kind of doing my best, in a kind of trance."

And then the ambulance arrived. Jed felt a brief sense of relief before a sobering realization set in: "I knew, I mean I could tell, moving me was going to be bad. I couldn't move and they were going to be moving the thing that really hurt, a lot. And then they started shuffling me around and lifted me up."

Jed remained fully conscious through the whole episode: "It was mind-bending pain. You know, like everything goes white. I think I probably howled quite a bit from there to St. Vincent's. That's where things start to fade, because of the pain, my consciousness started to fade."

The ambulance ride to St. Vincent's was short, and the ambulance was practically flying. Jed was screaming for pain medication. He had still not yet received anything to numb his agony. There was no time.

"I remember the EMT saying, 'Hold on, we'll get you something when we get to the hospital.'"

When they finally arrived at St. Vincent's, doctors surrounded Jed and immediately began questioning him. They needed details. Jed's response was clear: "Give me something for the pain, then I'll answer your questions."

He began to fade in and out. But one memory remains crystal clear: seeing his girlfriend, Megan. She had been at their apartment in Brooklyn when she received news of the accident. She went straight to the hospital.

"I remember Megan being there, worrying over me. It's such a hard memory. She looked so upset. She was in tears. I remember feeling helpless. I wanted to do something to convince her, you know, that I was going to be okay. I remember feeling really confident as they wheeled me into surgery, and I said to Megan, 'I'll see you on the other side.' And then they whisked me off."

That was the last thing Jed remembers of that night.

As Jed continued to bleed out in the operating room, orthopedic specialists busily debated how best to save his mangled leg. Then the lead vascular surgeon arrived. He immediately waved them off. As Jed pieced it together later, the vascular surgeon had said something to the effect of, "There is no way this man is going to live with you guys futzing about him. We've got to figure out a way to stop the bleeding." And then, Jed remembers, the surgeon basically booted the orthopedists out of the operating room.

Jed's condition was critical. How long it would take to put him back together was not yet clear. Nor was it clear that Jed's leg could be saved. He had no way of knowing that soon the doctors would be having conversations with Megan and with his immediate family to explain the severity of his injuries. And to prepare them for the very real possibility that he might not make it.

That first night in the trauma center, Jed was in surgery for hours. The medical team labored to keep him alive. As the severity of the assault to his body came into focus, it was decided that he was going to need multiple surgeries, and that the safest way to pull that off was to medically induce him into a coma. Three days after the accident, it became clear that Jed's leg could not be saved. The entire left leg was amputated. The hip joint was removed as well. Additional surgeries were planned. It looked like Jed was going to have to be kept in a coma for some time.

A medically induced coma is only vaguely like the kind of coma that results from an accident, such as when a traumatic head injury causes the brain to swell or when the brain is deprived of oxygen. A medically induced coma is brought on by intentional, controlled doses of barbiturates, usually pentobarbital or propofol. The barbiturates reduce brain metabolism and induce a temporary state of deep consciousness akin to anesthesia.

Although brain activity is reduced in medically induced comas, there is still some cognitive processing. Patients often report wild and vivid dreams. Sometimes these dreams incorporate sounds that are around them while they are comatose, or medical procedures or sensory experiences, such as being touched or moved.

In one indelible dream, Jed felt like he was falling. He was disembodied. Weightless. Falling endlessly. It was not a pleasant sensation.

"I was in an open-air car of some sort, a structure, like an airplane. Not a human body. I was falling, straight down, next to a waterfall. I was falling parallel to a waterfall. I was falling fast. Careening. It wasn't really like I was flying. I wasn't in control. It was kind of vague, but the salient part, the emotion, the physical sense, was a free fall, an endless free fall. It was awful.

"I don't know how long it went on, the falling, it just went on and on. It seemed like I had been falling for a very long time.

"And then . . . Whoosh. I sort of landed.

"It was pretty hard but it wasn't disruptive. It was like 'Oh, I am back in this body. I am not falling anymore, and I am back in my body.' It was over. I had been in a state of . . . what would you call it . . . limbo, and then I was back in myself.

"And then, this sounds kind of crazy, this medicine man that I had once met, at like a sweat lodge, his voice came to me. He said something like, 'You had a curse on you,' or 'Your family had a curse' . . . something like that . . . 'and now the debt is settled. Everything is going to be fine.'"

Jed laughed as he recalled the medicine man and referred to these kinds of dreams as "my weird psycho-spiritual dreams." In another dream, the famous chef Mario Batali visited him along with his business partner Joe Bastianich. Jed knew them both. They were Babbo's co-owners. Mario and Joe had, in fact, visited Jed in the hospital while he was comatose. He distinctly heard, or at least remembers hearing, his mother's voice announcing their arrival. But the meeting, in Jed's barbiturate-laden brain, took place not in a sterile hospital room but in a verdant field "somewhere in the South, like Virginia, in the springtime." Jed didn't recall any particular conversation, only Mario and Joe's presence and the peaceful setting.

The bucolic location was a common theme in Jed's coma dreams.

"I had this whole dream reality built around my convalescence in a plush, long-term care facility. There was a gazebo and rolling hills. The sun was shining. It was warm and pleasant."

The gazebo reminded Jed of a similar gazebo in the small town he grew up in. It appeared in several other dreams. He remembers dreaming of marrying Megan several times. The wedding dreams sometimes became quite bizarre.

"The first one," Jed recalls, "was really weird. My sister's boyfriend, now her husband, now my brother-in-law, was searching online, on the Korean underground, you know like the Internet underground, trying to find a vintage dress for Megan, like a Beatles 1960s-era vintage dress. And we were then driving around this circular mountain, winding up the road to a cupola, a gazebo on top. We were in a red sports car, a convertible. Megan was happy. It was all very early 60s vintage. A 60s vintage wedding.

"There weren't that many details of the wedding in the dream, but then I remember we had to repeat it. Megan's father was not happy about something in the wedding, so we had to do it all over again. We were married twice."

Jed's hospital dreams were usually odd, but some were profoundly disturbing. These often had a paranoid flavor and involved some sort of punishment for wrongdoing. He called these his "warped" dreams.

"Once I was stuck on a submarine for two weeks. Stuck cooking. I was the cook. It was the punishment for a bad deed, something like that. Like I had misbehaved and was being punished."

In another dream, Jed remembers being shaved by a nurse or orderly. This could easily have been a residue of an actual event, part of the actual preparation for surgery. But in the dream, Jed was watching the action from a distance. He was watching himself being shaved, and it was extremely painful. The nurse was punishing Jed deliberately.

"It was weird. There was this persecutory content, like I had been a bad boy, or something, I don't remember what they said, but clearly they were angry and they were punishing me."

In one of the worst dreams, he recalled, he was on a farm: "This was not a pleasant convalescent home. This was like a farm for . . . I want to say it was like a fat farm. It was terrible. Again, it was a facility somewhere in the South, a pleasant place. But the patients were just spilling over their beds. They're all . . . hideously overweight. It was terrible, almost like a *foie gras* farm for humans, but a hospital. They're all being fed intravenously. I was there in a bed, being fed. I was enormous. I was spilling over the bed too. I was farmed."

•

SURPRISINGLY LITTLE IS known about the mechanism behind such nightmarish imagery, or, for that matter, how often it occurs in induced comas. But it does seem that many patients who have been through induced comas do report these kinds of bizarre hallucinatory dreams.[1]

A common complaint is that the dreams are eerie and frightening. Some people describe feeling that they were surrounded by "beings" that were bad or dark or evil, and being taken to "all kinds of places" and experiencing "horrific things." The induced coma tends to render this nightmarish quality all the more disturbing simply because it can seem to be never ending. That's because induced comas can last a long time. And unlike the dreams we usually experience during the course of a normal night's sleep, coma dreams are not punctuated by cycles of sleeping and waking. The dreams a person might experience during a coma can go on and on. One former patient said it was like "an ongoing nightmare that I couldn't wake from." Another described "a nightmare that seemed to last forever . . . an endless series of terrible events, one situation leading to the next."

Something about the fact that the dreams just keep going makes them seem "unbelievably vivid and detailed," almost hyperreal. Many people who have experienced induced comas have reported that even after they were brought out of the coma, it still took them several days to realize that the dream events had not actually happened. Worse still, after returning to normal waking consciousness, many found that their coma-induced dreams wouldn't go away. They seemed to have left a haunting residue, not unlike a traumatic memory.

Another former patient said, "The nightmares I had while in a coma, they still continue to this day," adding that they "were and are still so real."

Some have complained that the dream memories are worse than the injuries that necessitated the coma in the first place. For example, "It was more difficult to get over the nightmares than to recover physically," and, "It took me *much* longer to heal from the imagery in that coma than it did the physical injuries."

It's not clear what to make of these kinds of retrospective memories because no one has ever systematically studied them. It may be that only people with the worst reactions will take the time to talk of their experiences. And in fact, not all coma survivors report nightmarish dreams. Some report that they do not remember any dreams at all from their comas.

Nonetheless, former intensive care unit (ICU) patients reported strikingly similar experiences in a recent study. Hallucinatory experiences are so common in ICUs—in part from the effects of psychoactive drugs—that there is a name for the phenomenon, *ICU psychosis*.[2] In the study, 88 percent of the patients interviewed reported having intrusive memories of the hallucinations and nightmares they had while in the ICU—which had included things like nurses turning patients into zombies, guns spouting blood, or birds laughing at each other. They also said that these images continued to invade their consciousness even months after their hospital release.

•

NONE OF THIS boded well for Jed. Not only did he suffer a ghastly traumatic event. Not only did he remember every detail of it: the wheels crushing his leg, the screaming, the bleeding, the icy pavement, the searing pain, the tears on Megan's face. Now, to pile it on further, he would also have indelible memories of bizarre "warped" coma dreams. And, if that were not enough, eventually the medical team would bring Jed out of the coma and he would discover that his entire leg, clean up to the hip, was gone.

Jed's family was worried. He had been in the coma for six long weeks. During that time, his body had been handled, rearranged, and patched together. He had endured almost twenty different surgeries. In addition to the amputation, he'd had a tracheotomy, and his colon had been rerouted. What would happen when he came to? What would he remember? How would he react to the knowledge that his leg had been amputated? How would they tell him? And how would he deal with the trauma of such a horrible ordeal?

To everyone's surprise, Jed already knew his leg was gone. He was not sure how he knew, but he knew. Maybe some of the discussion among the medical team penetrated the coma. Maybe somehow he felt or understood the medical procedures. Or maybe he just understood that the damage was too great.

"I had a sense that my leg was really messed up," Jed recalled, "like on the pavement. I could see it was bad. I was on death's door. So on some level I already knew. And for whatever reason, I woke up thinking that it was gone already. I was not surprised."

The process of bringing someone out of an induced coma happens gradually over the course of several days. This allows for the mind to relocate itself in place and time and for the brain to regain control of the body. It also helps to minimize the sudden shock of waking up in a strange place. Jed recalls becoming aware of his surroundings "in pieces." "I don't remember thinking anything like, 'Oh, here I am in the ICU.' Nothing like that," he said. "It was more gradual. There was a slow reckoning. I knew about the leg, but I remember looking down and seeing this hole in my abdomen, and then all these tubes, and all these scars."

Then there were adverse side effects to deal with: "I remember waking up and realizing I couldn't talk. Someone was there telling me I wouldn't be able to talk until the breathing tube was removed."

It was five days after waking before Jed would be able to talk again. During that time, he could communicate only through gestures or by writing short notes. The use of a breathing tube also meant that his throat had become extremely dry.

"One of the worst parts about waking up, one of the most aversive aspects of it, was that I was parched. My throat was dry as a bone. And they wouldn't allow me to drink anything. They have to clear you first to swallow. There is a whole swallow team that comes around."

Some of the first experiences Jed remembers after becoming conscious were comforting. He recalls a great desire to see Megan. He remembered "how soothing her presence was."

But soon the recollections became much more difficult. Jed began to come to grips with how he had lost his leg. Within a couple of days, he was flooded with memories of the accident.

"I was still not able to talk yet. Then I remember just being pummeled with these memories. I kept replaying the accident. The memories had a deep valence. You know, like a sort of deep traumatic valence. I thought, 'Oh wow! I can't believe I have to process all this!'"

The coma memories had also begun to plague him. These were just as bad, maybe worse.

"I spent more time trying to avoid the dream content. You know, it was so salient. There were these themes of paranoia, violation, punishment, mistrust of my environment. All really powerful."

And then, to Jed's amazement, it just stopped.

The intrusive images tapered off and then simply stopped. He could remember all the details of the accident. He could easily remember the vivid dreams. But after just a few days, these memories no longer invaded his consciousness. No flashbacks. No frightening images chasing him. He could bring them to mind if and when he wanted to, but he was also able to keep his mind clear when he wanted to.

"The memories were flooding me for the first couple of days for sure. But then they receded. You know, so quickly. I thought how funny that was, how the salience of those memories faded and I no longer had the type of intense reaction that I did when I first woke up."

For Jed, the transition was profound.

"I had burning questions. I was mostly wondering why I wasn't more messed up. I was really puzzled, you know. If everybody gets PTSD, why was I doing okay? That was my question, really. Why was I doing okay?"

•

WHY WAS JED doing okay?

How could anybody possibly be okay after such a horrific experience?

The question seems at once profound and unanswerable.

But there is an answer. We'll never know with absolute certainty, of course, why Jed was psychologically unscathed. The fact that he was in a coma for so long shrouds at least part of his experience in mystery. But we can explain the rest of it, not only for Jed but for anybody faced with serious adversity.

The story begins with how we think about trauma. According to a conventional view, Jed should have been psychologically overwhelmed, his seemingly rapid turnaround nothing more than an illusion, a short-lived denial of the more pernicious psychological wounds lurking deeper in the recesses of his mind. But this perspective, which has dominated our understanding for most of the past half-century, is woefully incomplete.

Until recently, most of what we have known about trauma came from the study of the most severe responses, such as post-traumatic stress disorder, or PTSD. It goes without saying that we should do everything we can to understand severe trauma. The problem arises when we focus only on that goal and ignore the experiences of those who don't show such extreme reactions. When that happens, we get to know a lot about what can go wrong but not much about what might go right. And, unfortunately, we slowly come to believe that things can only go wrong, that traumatic stress inevitably produces lasting trauma and PTSD.

This kind of reasoning is known as essentialism. It is rooted in the belief that a traumatic event is a "natural kind," that it has an immutable and unobservable *essence* that causes us to feel and behave in certain ways.[3] We tend to think of PTSD in this way. When we essentialize these concepts, we assume that humans did not invent or create them, but rather, that they always existed, and that humans simply discovered them. Essentialist assumptions are not necessarily wrong. A dog is different from a cat. A stone is different from water. But sometimes essentialist concepts miss the mark, especially when they pertain to mental states. And, as we will see shortly, the conventional view of trauma misses the mark by a wide margin. Neither trauma nor PTSD is a static, immutable category. They are dynamic states with fuzzy boundaries that unfold and change over time.

Yes, PTSD, or at least something like it, does happen. And, sadly, when it does happen, it is often debilitating. But an extreme reaction like PTSD does not simply come about instantaneously because of exposure to a trauma-inducing event. Violent or life-threatening events are undeniably difficult, and most people who encounter them experience at least some form of traumatic stress. They may feel stunned and anxious, for example, or struggle to manage disturbing thoughts, images, and memories. These reactions vary across people and events, and typically they are short-lived, lasting no more than a few hours or a few days, sometimes even a few weeks. In this transient form, traumatic stress is a perfectly natural response. But it is not PTSD.

PTSD is what happens when traumatic stress doesn't go away, when it festers and expands and eventually stabilizes into a more enduring state of distress. But this outcome is not nearly as common as we might think. Research over the past several decades has shown incontrovertibly that most people exposed to violent or life-threatening events do *not* develop PTSD. And that can only mean that the events themselves are not inherently traumatic. In fact, no event, not even a violent or life-threatening event, is inherently traumatic. Such events are only "potentially traumatic." A good part of the rest of it is up to us.

That "rest of it" varies a great deal more than the standard perspective on trauma supposes. Although most people do not develop PTSD, some still suffer in other ways. They may struggle with traumatic stress for a few months or longer, for example, before gradually recovering, or they may begin with less severe stress reactions that slowly worsen over time. Yet, even when we account for these diverse patterns, we still find that most people—a clear majority—are able to cope with traumatic stress reasonably well. Most people exposed to potentially traumatic events are able to continue on with their normal lives relatively quickly and without suffering *any* long-term difficulties. In short, most people are resilient. My own research has shown this repeatedly, in study after study. Research by other scientists has shown it, too. When we look across the full range of research that has been conducted—studies on all kinds of highly aversive or potentially traumatic events—resilience is almost always the most common outcome.

But even when we account for the empirical fact that we humans are highly resilient, we are still left with the even bigger question of why. Why, when horrible things happen, are we able to cope so well, to shake it off and get on with our lives? What is it that we do that allows us to be so resilient?

Ironically, this is where the failings of the conventional view of trauma are most glaring. If PTSD simply happens because of a traumatic event, then, by the same essentialist logic, most people are resilient to trauma simply because they are resilient. In other words, the conventional view leaves us no choice but to assume that there is something in resilient people, some essence, that makes them impervious.

Most formulations of resilience you are likely to come across are mired in this static essentialist reasoning. They tell us that resilience is about having the right qualities, the five or seven traits of highly resilient people. If you have the traits on the list, you are resilient. If you do not have them, you are not. The straightforwardness of this approach has an obvious appeal. It's clean and simple. And it leaves open the hopeful possibility that one can always try to develop these traits and eventually become resilient.

But a closer look reveals the flaw in this logic. The problem is not with the number of traits on the list. My own research has identified a good many characteristics that correlate with resilient outcomes. Eventually, no doubt, we'll find more. The number doesn't matter. The problem is that when we rely on a one-size-fits-all list of key traits of resilience, we always come up short. I call this the *resilience paradox*. We can identify statistical correlates of resilience—the so-called traits of resilient people—but paradoxically, when something aversive happens, these correlates don't actually tell us much about who will be resilient and who will not.

The reason is that resilience, like trauma, is a moving target. The stress induced by a potentially traumatic event unfolds over time. It shifts and changes even as we struggle to manage it. These events also tend to impact our lives, often in ways that create new stresses and new problems. They may, for example, cause physical injury, or temporary loss of a job or housing. It takes time to adapt to these impacts. And it takes more than a simple set of fixed traits.

Abundant research has shown us, in fact, that no one trait, or even set of traits, is ever always effective. As we'll see later, literally any trait, any behavior we might think of, has both benefits and costs. Simply put, what works in one situation at one point in time may not work as well, or may even be harmful, in another situation or at another point in time. Even traits and behaviors that seem most obviously useful—say, expressing emotion, or seeking support from others—aren't universally helpful. And in some situations, traits and behaviors that we typically think of as problematic, such as suppressing emotion, are exactly what we need. This means, effectively, that we have to work out the best solution moment by moment as we struggle, and then we have to readjust as we go along. In other words, we have to be flexible.

Although it sounds simple, there is a lot to this kind of flexibility. And because it plays such a key role in how we adapt to adversity, I will devote a good part of this book to breaking it down. For starters, flexibility is not a passive process. Potentially traumatic events are painful and disturbing, and typically we want nothing more than to push them out of our thoughts. Adapting to such events requires that we think, actively and systematically, about what we are experiencing and why. And to do that effectively, we need to be motivated and engaged. We need what I call a *flexibility mindset*.

Once we have that mindset, that conviction, in place, then we can move on to the nuts and bolts of meeting the challenge. This gets us into a series of steps I call *the flexibility sequence*. As we cycle through these steps, we work out what is happening to us and what we can do to manage it. There is also a crucial corrective step where we determine whether a strategy we chose is working or we should change to another strategy. Together, these steps allow us to flexibly utilize the tools we have, whatever traits and behaviors and resources we might have at our disposal, so that we can more effectively adapt and move forward. It is important to point out that these are not rare abilities. They are simply underappreciated features of the human mind, and they can be nurtured and improved.

When I give public lectures on these ideas, invariably someone will tell me that it is hard to believe the conventional wisdom about trauma could possibly be so wrong. Perhaps you are thinking the same thing. If so, that's not surprising. After all, many of the ideas I've just described may run counter to what you have been told for most of your life. And, of course, it would be inaccurate to say that the conventional view is completely unfounded. That view, and, in particular, the concept of PTSD, was an indispensable step on the long road to understanding trauma. But we are now much farther along that road. And, as we'll see shortly, the insights and evidence we've picked up along the way leave little doubt that the conventional perspective is simply no longer viable.

In the coming chapters, we will set the pieces in place for a new and more coherent framework, one that not only accounts for different trauma outcomes, such as resilience and PTSD, but also explains how those different outcomes develop. We'll delve deeply into the questions and ideas that led to that new perspective, and we'll take a good look at some of the research behind it. As we move forward, we won't forget about Jed. We'll check back in with him at various points in the book, and we'll also hear stories of other people who've struggled with serious adversity. But before we do all that, we need to start at the beginning. We need to go back in time to when humans first tried to make sense of trauma.

PART I

Two-Thirds

CHAPTER 1

The Invention of PTSD

There is a haunting diorama in New York's Museum of Natural History within the Hall of Human Origins. It is large. If it were possible to climb into it, a person could easily stand up and walk around. It's also exceptionally lifelike.

The lighting is intentionally dim. It takes a bit of time for the eyes to adjust. The first thing you notice is that at least one of the figures in the display, one closest to the glass, has a humanlike appearance. He looks like a small, early human ancestor. He is naked, and he is crouching.

The diorama portrays a scene from the Pleistocene era, something like a million years ago, maybe longer. The figure is *Homo erectus*. His hands are cupped and he is bent over a small stream, pausing to take a drink. His hairy, naked body looks relaxed. The stream is at the bottom of a hill and it is dusk. The water must have been refreshing.

As your eyes adjust further, you begin to make out other figures. You notice what appear to be animals. A pack of animals. Hyenas. They are alert, ears up, and approaching our ancestor from behind.

As you look closer at one of the hyenas, you can now see from his posture that he is in an attack crouch. He looks menacing. The silhouette of another hyena comes into focus. This one is closer, much closer: crouching, snout forward, ears back, most definitely preparing to attack. Prehistoric hyenas were big, and they were formidable predators. Our ancestor seems to be completely unaware of what is about to hit him. There is no sign of a weapon. He seems to have let down his guard. With a start, you realize that he's almost certain to meet a gruesome fate.

And if he somehow managed to survive the attack? Would he have been plagued by flashbacks? Frightening images of rushing animals. Gnashing teeth. Growling. Fighting, running, blood, and pain. Would he have been haunted by constant thoughts of the encounter? Suffered invasive memories and nightmares?

We will never know. All we have of the Pleistocene era is fossilized bones and other archeological clues that have allowed us to piece together only some aspects of life in the past. There is no written word. No artwork. No recorded thoughts or experiences.

It wasn't until much later, a period only around forty thousand years ago, that humans first began to represent their experiences in small statues and cave paintings. Among the most common subjects depicted in those early works of art were animals, hunting parties, and weapons. Clearly this was a dominant preoccupation. Humans were vulnerable, and life was dangerous. But around that same time, humans were also beginning to turn the tables. They were beginning to defend themselves and shift the survival balance. The prey was slowly becoming the predator.

But was there psychological trauma? Hunting and weapons mean danger. That's clear. But how do you depict trauma in a cave painting? We can draw weapons and a hunt or an attack. But trauma is a psychological response that is most easily conveyed in words. And that means we must travel forward even closer to our current era. It was only about five thousand years ago, in fact, that humans first began to develop written languages. At this point we might expect that for the first time we would begin to find mention of some sort of enduring psychological trauma. If not five thousand years ago, then sometime soon thereafter.

But when we look to that written legacy, the five thousand years or so of recorded language, we discover something truly remarkable. The concept of psychological trauma seems to be a surprisingly modern idea.

The Time Before Trauma

Among the earliest written texts, one of the most likely places we would expect to find mention of psychological trauma would be Homer's epic poem about the Trojan War, the *Iliad*. The poem was likely developed through years of oral tradition.[1] It was eventually written down, probably for the first time somewhere around 1000 BCE. Much of the story is mythical, but it's a narrative rooted in the details of an actual war between the Mycenaeans and the Hittites, more commonly remembered as "the Trojans," that had taken place many centuries earlier. The *Iliad* didn't pull punches, so to speak. The battle scenes were described in vivid detail. Warriors were wounded, maimed, and killed. And in the narrative accounts, there is no shortage of fear, anguish, dread, and courage. Both sides suffered devastating losses. They wept bitter tears. They wailed and they moaned. And despite the fact that each side remained in close proximity to the other, the soldiers made no attempt to hide their tormented grief.

Psychiatrist Jonathan Shay found such descriptions strikingly similar to stories of "toxic combat experiences" he had heard from modern soldiers in the Vietnam War.[2] Yet, as Shay pointed out, Homer gave no voice whatsoever to the presumed emotional trauma the Greeks and Trojans might have felt when the war had concluded.[3] Grief, yes. There were numerous descriptions of the intense grief experienced by soldiers for their fallen comrades, and by friends and families of those who would not return. But postwar traumatic reactions such as nightmares or intrusive flashbacks were simply not mentioned.

There are many other historical accounts that also describe harrowing incidents that today we would have no trouble labeling traumatic. But for the most part, again, these accounts never mentioned the words for "trauma" or "traumatic." Nor did they describe anything like the symptoms we now associate with PTSD. The idea that a dangerous or frightening event might cause lasting psychological difficulties does not appear in recorded history, literally anywhere, until relatively recently.

Only a very few historical accounts suggest anything even remotely like enduring psychological trauma. One of the most famous, and perhaps the first ever recorded, is a scene from Shakespeare's *Henry IV*, written sometime in the late sixteenth century. In one brief passage, the queen, Lady Percy, worries about the king's deteriorating mental condition at the hand of what seem to be war-induced nightmares and preoccupations. Whether these troubles might qualify as genuine PTSD symptoms is hard to say. Beyond this brief passage, neither Lady Percy nor the king mentions the topic again.

A less ambiguous account, written in the first person, emerged in the seventeenth century in the diaries of British aristocrat Samuel Pepys (pronounced *peeps*). Pepys was an intellectual, a confidant of King Charles II, and a friend to Isaac Newton. He lived a notable life, accrued a vast library of books, and accomplished a great many things. But he is remembered primarily for his diaries. For ten eventful years, Pepys dutifully recorded his thoughts and activities, observations about his friends, the court, and the events of the day, and then carefully stowed them away.

That Pepys's diary might mention trauma reactions when other sources were silent on the subject is probably no accident. Pepys was not making public disclosures. He wrote in archaic English and used a shorthand code, and, as far as is known, never circulated the diaries during his lifetime. After his death, his vast book collection, and with it the diaries, was donated to Cambridge University. There they languished, apparently untouched for over a century, until they were eventually discovered, decoded, and published.

One of the more significant passages from Pepys's journal describes the great fire that devastated London in 1666. Pepys was awakened in the middle of the night by signs of flames at some distance, but he assumed it was not serious and returned to bed. The next day, to his great shock, he found that the blaze had raged throughout the night, destroying hundreds of houses. He surveyed the damage, first from the vantage point of the Tower of London and then by boat. As the fire showed no signs of letting up, he rushed off to share this intelligence with the court.

Pepys roughed it throughout the emergency about as much as a seventeenth-century aristocrat might rough anything. It was a deeply trying time. He slept little and ate only sporadically. He busied himself with the considerable tasks of seeing that his household, his vast collection of precious books, and of course his gold, were relocated to places of safety. Pepys's business interests and courtly duties demanded, however, that he also regularly survey the appalling progress of the blaze. He did this by boat when he could, but mostly on foot.

"Our feet ready to burn, walking through the towne among the hot coals," he complained.

Although he maintained the demeanor of the poised diarist, Pepys did not shrink from recording the anguish he felt at the hands of such devastation. He was frequently brought to tears and at times overcome with fear. In one passage, he noted "how horridly the sky looks, all on a fire in the night. Was enough to put us out of our wits, and indeed, it was extremely dreadful, for it looks just as if it was at us, and the whole of heaven on fire."

After five long days, most of the blaze had finally abated. But Pepys's experiences stayed with him. On the last night of the fire, he wrote that he "slept pretty well, but still had a fear of fire in my heart." Several months later he was still "mightily troubled the most of the night with fears of fire, which I cannot get out of my head to this day."[4] Half a year later, Pepys shared his surprise at finding that he was still haunted during the night.

"It is strange to think how, to this very day, I cannot sleep at night without great terrors of fire, and this very night I could not sleep till almost two in the morning through thoughts of fire."[5]

Finding Trauma

Pepys never used the word "trauma." According to the *Oxford English Dictionary*, although the term was in circulation in the seventeenth century, it was reserved at that time exclusively for describing an acute physical insult in the field of medicine. Even references to physical trauma did not appear with any frequency until the mid-nineteenth century. By that time, the industrial revolution was in full swing, and with it a marked increase in the frequency of industrial accidents causing serious injury. Nineteenth-century physicians treating the survivors of those accidents occasionally noted odd behaviors or mysterious, unexplainable symptoms. But it was believed that such symptoms were due to an underlying physical cause, even if that physical cause had not yet been detected.

Probably the most famous example of mid-nineteenth-century attitudes about trauma is the concept of *railway spine*, a condition proposed by a Danish physician, John Eric Erichsen.[6] At the time, new railways were proliferating throughout the Western world. But the early days of rail travel were, to put it bluntly, pretty nasty. Trains were dirty, noisy, and most of all, dangerous. Outrageously violent accidents were not uncommon, and there was little protection from injury when they occurred. Railway cars were flimsy, with wooden frames and few safeguards. The results were often gruesome.

Increasingly, rail travelers who had experienced even minor accidents were reporting to their doctors strange and oddly psychological symptoms, including memory difficulties, lack of appetite, nightmares, perceptual confusion, anxiety, and inexplicable fatigue and irritability. Typically, and most perplexing, they often showed no detectable signs of any physical insult. Erichsen's infamous explanation of this problem was that these patients were suffering from microlesions of the spine—minute, and essentially undetectable, abrasions to the spinal cord that were jumbling signals to their brains and wreaking havoc in their emotional lives.

Erichsen's ideas were hotly debated. But his attempts to sway a skeptical medical community were not made any easier by his admission that some of the patients showing signs of railway spine might have been malingering as a ploy to gain compensation from the railway. In what is probably more than a striking coincidence, this same period also witnessed the creation of liability insurance.[7]

Whether they were to be believed or not, survivors of industrial accidents kept showing up in doctors' offices to recount their odd symptoms. Some of those survivors made their way to eminent neurologist Hermann Oppenheim's Berlin office. Oppenheim gradually came to believe that these strange symptoms were due to more than physical trauma, that they bespoke an underlying psychological problem. In 1889, he proposed his controversial thesis in a book titled *Die Traumatischen Neurosen* (The traumatic neuroses).[8] The book had little lasting impact; indeed, few people outside of those interested in the history of ideas remember Oppenheim. Regardless, he had made his mark. His 1889 book still stands today as the first medical use of the term *trauma* to describe a purely psychological response.

Shell Shock

As the idea of psychological trauma slowly simmered, the world moved into the twentieth century. Then the heat was turned up. Europe was soon engulfed in a massive war, aptly remembered as World War I. It was by any account an absolutely terrible war, dominated by vast, deadly, and ultimately futile trench warfare campaigns. The death toll was staggering. And when soldiers who had managed to survive the carnage eventually returned to their homelands, many seemed oddly changed: not quite able to get over what they had been through, not quite capable of describing what it was that was troubling them.

World War I forced a new explanatory term into daily parlance: *shell shock*. The term unambiguously described a mental rather than a purely physical breakdown. But inherent in the term was also clear evidence of the lingering ambivalence surrounding the idea of trauma. The word "shock" suggests intensity but also a transient state, something that should naturally abate in a relatively short time. Distressed soldiers, it was assumed, would simply "get over it." The word also carries an unmistakably suspicious, if not insulting, tone. What was the real cause behind this kind of disability? Was it just plain weakness? Or worse, cowardice and malingering?

These suspicions were not harmless, especially for the soldiers who endured them. As the war dragged on through stalemate and bitter winters, thousands of cases of shell shock were recorded. In the harsh reality of the trenches, however, they were often dismissed. Soldiers complaining of psychological problems were ignored, disbelieved, or worse, punished, often severely. Hundreds of soldiers were executed—infamously "shot at dawn"—for cowardice. Some had deserted; some had refused to follow orders, or were simply unable to follow them. But undoubtedly, many were genuinely suffering from combat trauma.

Twenty-five-year-old British private Henry Farr was one of them. After fighting in the trenches for two exhausting years, practically without respite, Farr was ordered to the front lines in the Battle of the Somme. The Somme offensive was one of the largest and bloodiest engagements of the war, dragging on for almost five months and producing staggering carnage. More than a million soldiers were killed or injured at the site. Farr had had enough. He was exhausted and refused to return to the front. His superiors would have none of it. They charged him with "misbehaving before the enemy in such a manner as to show cowardice" and ordered him to face court-martial. Unwisely, he chose to represent himself during the hearing. The trial took only twenty minutes. He was executed the next day.[9]

In hindsight, with almost a century of advances into psychological trauma behind us, these actions seem barbarous. They did to the soldiers' families as well. For decades, friends and relatives of the executed soldiers fought to correct the historical record. It wasn't until 2006, almost ninety years after the war's end, that many of these soldiers were finally posthumously pardoned.

Henry Farr's daughter, Gertrude, lived long enough to see her father's name cleared.

"I have always argued," she said, "that my father's refusal to rejoin the frontline . . . was in fact the result of shellshock, and I believe that many other soldiers suffered from this, not just my father."[10]

The Scary Parts

When World War I ended in 1918, an enormous sigh of relief rose over Europe. The war had been one of the bloodiest and most lethal in recorded history, and the public was more than happy to let the idea of shell shock recede into the background. The only problem was that it refused to go away.

One reason, surprisingly enough, was poetry. Many of the young British intellectual elite had fought in the war, including a new generation of poets. Until that time, war poetry had always been a patriotic form, romanticizing the bonds of soldiery and praising the unsurpassed honor of giving one's life in the service of one's country.

At the onset of World War I, one of the new generation of poets, Wilfred Owen, was still able to echo that sentiment:

> *O meet it is and passing sweet*
> *To live in peace with others,*
> *But sweeter still and far more meet*
> *To die in war for brothers.*[11]

But Owen and his poems were soon to undergo a dramatic transformation. Owen had enlisted in the British officers corps. He trained for seven months and then found himself on his way overseas. Initially, his letters home had been jovial. But reality quickly set in. Owen had been sent to the front, directly into the ongoing carnage of the Battle of the Somme. He confessed his horror in letters to his mother, writing, "I can see no excuse for deceiving you about these last four days. I have suffered seventh hell."

Death and destruction were everywhere. But the worst part, for Owen, was "the universal pervasion of ugliness!"

"Hideous landscapes, vile noises, foul language and nothing but foul, even from one's own mouth (for all are devil ridden), everything unnatural, broken, blasted; the distortion of the dead, whose unburiable bodies sit outside the dug-outs all day, all night, the most execrable sights on earth," he wrote. "In poetry we call them the most glorious. But to sit with them all day, all night . . . and a week later to come back and find them still sitting there, in motionless groups, THAT is what saps the 'soldierly spirit.'"

Owen was sent to an advance post: "not at the front," as he put it, but "in front of it." He had been sent into "no man's land," the barren dead space between the barbed wire and the trenches of the warring sides.

"The Germans," Owen told his mother, "knew we were staying there and decided we shouldn't."

The Germans shelled the area repeatedly. To conceal their presence, Owen and twenty-five other men packed themselves tightly into a dugout, essentially a large hole in the ground. A shell had exploded near one of the openings to the dugout, closing it off. Escaping by the other opening was impossible. They had no choice but to wait it out. And as they waited, their hiding place gradually filled with several feet of water.

"Those fifty hours were the agony of my happy life. I nearly broke down and let myself drown in the water that was now slowly rising over my knees," Owen later wrote.

"I did not wash my face, nor take off my boots, nor sleep a deep sleep. For twelve days we lay in holes, where at any moment a shell might put us out."

Then one of those shells struck close, just a few yards from Owen's sleeping head. He was blown into the air and clear out of the dugout. Somehow, he managed to find protection in another hole, one "just big enough to lie in," and covered himself with a piece of corrugated tin that he had found. The worst of it for Owen, however, was that one of his fellow officers, Second Lieutenant Hubert Gaukroger, was blown out of the hole with him. But Gaukroger was not so lucky. He didn't survive. His mangled, lifeless body lay nearby, half buried with earth.

Owen was trapped in that spot, with Gaukroger's corpse, for several days. When he was finally discovered and relieved by his company, "he was found to be confused, trembling, and behaving strangely."[12]

The event had pushed him over the edge.

"You know it was not the Bosche [Germans] that worked me up, nor the explosives," he wrote. "It was living so long by poor old Cock Robin, as we used to call Second Lieutenant Gaukroger, who lay not only nearby, but in various places around and about, if you understand. I hope you don't!"

Owen had been in the conflict only four months. He was diagnosed with shell shock and sent to a hospital in Scotland to recuperate.

It was in Scotland that he penned his now famous war poems. But in the new poems, Owen had exchanged his formerly romantic depictions of the brotherhood of soldiers for far darker visions of the hellish nature of war. He wrote of nightmares, of dead soldiers who held out their hands to take him with them, and of the pitiless faces of the dying, which he could not make go away.[13]

Owen could have remained in Great Britain for the duration of the war. But after a period of respite, he volunteered to return to the front. He was on a mission. He had found his voice and he felt it was his moral duty to write of the soldier's experience.

Sadly, his return ended tragically. Just days before the war's end, he was killed in battle. His mother received the bitter news in a telegram on Armistice Day.

It was another great war poet, Siegfried Sassoon, who made sure Owen's poems were published. They had a powerful impact at the time and are remembered to this day, not only for their lyrical, gritty realism but also for their unprecedented sympathy for the plight of the soldier.[14]

As moving as Owen's poems might be, admittedly they are not pulp fiction. Poetry was then, and it remains, a relatively refined literary format, an acquired taste. As is often the case, though, a far more accessible account of the emotional pain of war was soon to follow. In 1928, Erich Maria Remarque published his now famous novel *All Quiet on the Western Front*. It offered a gripping fictional account of the psychological toll of trench warfare and of the difficulties of returning to civilian life. The novel quickly became a runaway best seller.

Inventing PTSD

World War I had devastated Europe. But postwar territorial solutions quickly frayed into renewed political tension, and, in just two decades, the world was again at war. This time it was even worse. Technology had advanced, as had war tactics, and with these changes came new ways to suffer. And again, psychological casualties surfaced as an unwelcome but unavoidable topic.

By the time of World War II, ideas about trauma had advanced slightly. On the positive side, the actions of traumatized soldiers were no longer seen as acts of cowardice deserving of punishment. But the model had changed to a psychological one, and war trauma was now considered a sign of inherent psychological weakness. The term *neurosis* was often used to describe it. Even more troubling, trauma was thought to be a temporary, short-lived problem that could be alleviated with a little rest.

World War II also resulted in the inaugural publication, in the United States, of the *Diagnostic and Statistical Manual of Mental Disorders*. This was the first version of what is now commonly known as the DSM, the bible of mental disorders. The first version, the DSM-I, included a vague quasi-trauma diagnosis: *gross stress reaction*. As with most disorders in the DSM-I, there were no formal criteria or list of symptoms. Gross stress reaction was distinguished from other forms of mental illness only because it was thought to be transient and reversible. Tellingly, the DSM-I advised that if gross stress reaction continued, the diagnosis should be discarded in favor of other, more definitive maladies that might capture the deeper underlying problem.

World War II lasted six long years and again resulted in sweeping devastation. The United States played a significant role in the second half of the war and then quickly became embroiled in other wars that followed—starting with the conflict in Korea in 1950. The stream of psychological casualties flowed on. A second DSM was published in 1968, DSM-II, and eventually gross stress reaction was replaced by an equally vague diagnosis, *adjustment reaction to adult life*. Not much had changed. The new diagnosis still lacked a formal criterion for trauma reactions, and it retained the lingering assumption that the problem was only a transient disturbance.

The 1960s and 1970s brought sweeping political and cultural change. Probably the two most significant factors influencing how trauma was perceived were the Vietnam War and the rapid evolution of television. The seemingly endless Vietnam War was exceedingly unpopular, and as it dragged on the country found itself embroiled in protest and political tension. Against this backdrop, war casualties became part of the national discourse. And this time, those casualties, and the horror of war, were televised, brought directly into American homes on the nightly news. Soon those nightly images were given flesh by the many returning soldiers who found themselves unable to function or rejoin society. Treatment providers found themselves at a loss. They clamored for a solution, or at least a diagnosis that would help them identify those most in need.

Then, finally, in 1980, several years after the war's end, the DSM-III was published, and with it, for the first time, a set of formal diagnostic criteria for enduring psychological trauma reactions. This was post-traumatic stress disorder, PTSD. It was unlike any of its predecessors. The PTSD diagnosis did not assume that the disorder was transient and reversible, or that it was due to cowardice or to inner weakness. Rather, PTSD was viewed as a disease that developed in response to horrific events that almost anyone would find distressing.

The symptoms of PTSD were organized into several different subcategories. One of the most prominent sets of features revolved around intrusive memories—sudden, involuntary, and highly unpleasant memories that repeatedly force their way into consciousness as painful reminders of the details of the traumatic event. Like

Pepys's haunting recollections of the London fire, these intrusive memories often appear as vivid dreams or nightmares. But they are most troublesome when they invade normal waking life. They can come on so suddenly and so intensely that they create the sensation, at least temporarily, that the trauma is happening all over again. Colloquially, we call these experiences *flashbacks*, because when they occur, they seem as real as the event itself, and just as disconcerting.

Intrusive memories can be triggered out of the blue by an otherwise harmless word, or a sound or an image that somehow serves as a reminder of a traumatic event. But once activated, they can be extremely difficult to manage. In the language of neuroscience, this problem is a "globally diminished capacity to use contextual information to modulate fear expression."[15] More plainly, even though it might be perfectly obvious that someone is in a safe environment, far removed from the original trauma—say, sitting in a chair at home or in a restaurant, or perhaps strolling on a quiet street—the rush of intrusive memories may seem all too real. The memories override the "contextual information" of the person's surroundings, and the past becomes the present. PTSD sufferers attempt to control these unbidden memories by avoiding people or places they know will remind them of the incident. More often than not, it doesn't do much good.

The randomness of the intrusions causes a heightened state of arousal, the feeling of being keyed up and constantly "on guard," as if danger might lurk just around the corner. As the desire to avoid the eliciting effects intensifies, the experience spirals into an increasingly debilitating cycle of intrusions and avoidance, intrusions and avoidance, intrusions and avoidance.

It is exhausting. Not surprisingly, people with PTSD are often irritable. They find it increasingly difficult to concentrate. Sleep has long ago failed to serve its restorative function. There is no respite, only a continual sense of foreboding and fear, sometimes guilt or anger, the feeling of being detached, alienated, and empty.

An Arbitrary and Expanding Diagnosis

The creation of the PTSD diagnosis unleashed a whirlwind of activity. Mental health professionals working on the front lines had for years argued that psychological trauma was real. The PTSD diagnosis meant they could finally say so, formally and officially. They wasted little time. New treatment programs began to appear almost overnight. Researchers dug in, too, quickly creating assessment instruments to better identify the disorder and to track its course and vicissitudes.

But right from the beginning, there were serious problems. For starters, the PTSD diagnosis is based on a medical disease model. A physical disease stems from a biological problem, usually an infectious pathogen or genetic abnormality, that can be verified by a physical test, such as a brain scan or blood assay. The symptoms of the disease are caused by that biological problem, and thus the symptoms help explain the disease. Psychological problems don't lend themselves well to a disease model. There is no clear pathogen or biological event that causes most mental disorders, including PTSD, and there is no physical test that can confirm its existence. To the contrary, severe trauma is a psychological reaction to the experience of an external and potentially traumatic event. There may be physical vulnerabilities that leave people susceptible to developing PTSD, but there is no clear physical cause that explains how or why the disorder comes about.[16]

A disease model of PTSD carries a rigid essentialist assumption that people either have the disorder or they don't. There is no in-between. The problem here is that psychological problems, including the reactions people have to potentially traumatic events, tend not to fall into neat categories. We can invent categories. That's easy. But inventing a category doesn't mean it actually exists in nature. For example, we commonly think of people as young, middle-aged, old, and so on. But there are no inherent categories in aging. Age is simply a continually increasing number. The same is true for PTSD symptoms. People exposed to potentially traumatic events can experience a wide range of symptoms. Some have only a few of these symptoms, some have many of them, and some have most or all of them. The symptoms make the most sense as a continuum. Statistical analyses show that there is no coherent point, no latent or emergent category, that clearly marks when the disorder is present or absent. This turns out to be the case, actually, for most mental disorders.[17]

These problems arise in part because mental health disorders are not created empirically. They are essentially invented by committee: by groups of experts who debate and argue, sometimes for months or even years, until they finally come to an agreement about what a disorder should look like. The process can be quite convoluted, more a compromise between warring factions than a consensus, and can produce some pretty complicated and heterogeneous diagnoses. The PTSD diagnosis, with its various subcategories, is one of the most complicated and heterogeneous diagnoses out there. Several years ago, my colleagues Isaac Galatzer-Levy and Richard Bryant examined all the possible symptom combinations a person could have and still qualify for PTSD. For an earlier version of the diagnosis, they found close to 80,000 different symptom combinations. But for the most recent version, the PTSD diagnosis currently in use today, the number of possible symptom combinations soared to a whopping 636,120. This means, literally, that 636,120 people could each have a unique set of symptoms and still qualify for the same PTSD diagnosis.[18]

Even if we put these worrisome conceptual problems aside, there was still another difficulty uniquely tied to PTSD. As use of the diagnosis spread, it turned out that determining who had—or who might develop—the disorder was surprisingly difficult to pin down. This problem had to do with the fact that the PTSD diagnosis requires exposure to a prior traumatic event. In the original 1980 diagnosis, the definition of a trauma was intentionally narrow, encompassing only those events that could be considered "outside the range of usual human experience and that would be markedly distressing to almost anyone." But over the years, as the diagnosis spread to common use, mental health professionals began to feel that they were missing cases. They argued that the criteria were too narrow, and that more people suffered from PTSD than the definition captured. Trauma reactions, they concluded, were not the same for everyone. What was merely difficult and unpleasant for some people might be traumatic for others, and those people deserved the diagnosis and the option for treatment too.

These arguments eventually won the day. In subsequent versions of the DSM, the definition of a traumatic event was broadened to include a much wider array of potentially distressing experiences. This newly expanded definition was unquestionably effective in allowing more people to receive the diagnosis. But unfortunately, the revised phrasing initiated a maddening problem, one that remains unsolved to this day. By introducing subjectivity into the definition, the criteria became so ambiguous that practically anything extremely unpleasant could qualify as a trauma.[19]

PTSD Everywhere

Not everyone was thrilled with the newly expanded version of PTSD. In a review of the trauma field published in the prestigious *Annual Review of Psychology*, Harvard psychologist Richard McNally disparaged the expansion as "conceptual bracket creep."[20] Trauma specialist Gerald Rosen complained that the wider criteria opened up the possibility that even the expectation of future trauma could lead to PTSD, thus creating the "conceptual equivalent of 'pretraumatic' stress disorder" and moving the PTSD diagnosis a step closer to becoming meaningless.[21]

But the ever-expanding diagnosis was more than an academic or clinical question, and it has sent ripples out of the clinic and into our daily lives. For the first time in recorded history, the world began to talk about PTSD openly. Media and news reports regularly featured the all-too-real stories of soldiers who were not quite able to get their minds to let go of the war; of assault victims frozen by memories of their assailant; of hurricane survivors helplessly reliving the same dreadful moments when they were caught in the height of the storm; of survivors of motor vehicle accidents who were still riveted to attention by the sound of screeching tires or a blaring siren.

These stories are almost impossible to ignore. We are wired to detect and respond to threat—it's part of our biological inheritance—and when we hear these stories, we have to listen. Although we no longer run around naked like our ancient ancestor in the Museum of Natural History, in many ways we are still very much like him: pausing for a drink of water, unawares, with a pack of aggressive predators lurking in the distance. True, daily life seems much safer now. But we are not invulnerable and we know it. Dreadful things can and still do happen: violent injuries, assaults, disasters. By even the most conservative estimates, most people experience at least one such event during the course of their lifetime. Often more.[22] Stories of PTSD shout this to us. They warn us of the dangers out there, and of the consequences that await us should we let down our guard.

With so much attention on PTSD, it seems we have dramatically overcorrected. What was in the days of Samuel Pepys a hidden malady, shameful and confusing, to be admitted only in the coded text of a private diary, has now become the siren song of the twenty-first century. Trauma is no longer unspoken. It now boldly asserts itself in the name of a television series and in an online video game.[23] It is the subject of web pages and blogs.[24] It's in the names of professional organizations and scholarly journals. "Trauma" has become a part of the fabric of our daily lives, and its presence only seems to be growing. As journalist David Morris put it, trauma behaves "almost as if it were a virus, a pathogen content to do nothing besides replicate itself in the world over and over until only it remains," until it seems as if "PTSD is everywhere."[25] A provocative statement, to be sure, but where does the truth lie? And with all this PTSD, where or what is resilience?

CHAPTER 2

Finding Resilience

The idea of resilience didn't begin with potentially traumatic events. It wasn't horrific motor vehicle accidents, or violent assaults, or even the casualties of war. It wasn't even humans.

It was trees.

In the early 1970s, environmental ecologist Crawford Stanley "Buzz" Holling first began using the word "resilience" to describe how forests and other ecological systems managed to endure for long periods despite constant threats to their survival.[1] Holling emphasized that resilient systems, such as forests, are often beset by random and unpredictable events: things like fires or dramatic increases in insect populations. These random events impact the size and health of the forest. Yet, although a forest may appear to be unstable, that instability is actually part of how the system survives. For example, although fires can incur serious damage—they may reduce the forest's density and range—over the long term fires provide forests with a great many benefits. They clear ground-level brush. They allow more sunlight and water to reach younger trees, and the proliferation of new vegetation means more food for animals and for useful insect populations. Fires can also nourish the soil, remove old or weak trees, and help kill off disease or harmful insects. Some trees have even evolved to depend on fire as part of their reproductive cycle.

Not long after Holling began to write about the resilience of forests, the idea of resilience also began to appear in the literature on child development.[2] Theorists and researchers concerned with the welfare of disadvantaged children had begun to notice that a surprisingly large number of disadvantaged children seemed to be able to weather the ups and downs of their challenging circumstances and eventually managed to lead normal, healthy lives.

Early on, human resilience research tended to focus primarily on the kinds of problems that were likely to impede long-term development: things like poverty or chronic maltreatment or deprivation.[3] Studying these problems necessitated the use of a long-range lens. A lack of economic resources, for example, often leads to a self-perpetuating cycle of disadvantages.[4] Poverty and poor nutrition contribute to early school dropout and conduct problems, which in turn limits job opportunities, which in turn feeds back into the ongoing cycle of poverty. Similarly, maltreatment and abuse can devastate a young child's view of the world and his or her sense of self-esteem and trust. These deficits can then lead to social withdrawal, isolation, or violent and reckless behavior, which often leads to further victimization and self-harm later in life.[5]

Despite these seemingly debilitating conditions, developmental researchers found that children are surprisingly resilient. Sizable numbers of disadvantaged children consistently achieved normative developmental milestones. As adults they were able to experience healthy social relationships, for example, and to function competently in their jobs and in many other domains of normal adult life.[6]

This was startling news. And not surprisingly, the media took notice. Feature stories began to appear describing the discovery of "invincible" and "invulnerable" children, or the rare species of "superkids."[7] But although anyone who survives such disadvantages deserves all the accolades they might receive, these terms are highly misleading. Children who beat the odds are not invincible. They are not invulnerable. They are not superkids. And they are not nearly as rare as these phrases imply.

One of the pioneers of this research, Ann Masten, perhaps put it best: "The biggest surprise that emerged from the study of children who overcome adversity . . . was the *ordinariness* of the phenomenon."[8] To describe the commonplace nature of childhood adaptation to hardship, she coined the beautifully poetic phrase *ordinary magic*.[9] Not all children exposed to chronic adversities fare so well, of course. But as Masten and others have demonstrated, more children manage to thrive in such contexts than conventional wisdom suggested.

Expected to Overwhelm

The research on disadvantaged children provided strong evidence for the capacity of the human mind to overcome caustic circumstances. But what about more acute events, isolated and potentially traumatic ones that occurred against a backdrop of normal daily life? Curiously, despite the mounting evidence that children could thrive in a context of chronic deprivation, there was almost no interest in resilience after potential trauma. Almost everyone, including experts on human development, assumed that acute life-threatening events were in a category all by themselves. When faced with "conditions of extreme threat or in the immediate aftermath of a disaster," the experts concluded, "no one is expected to maintain a high-level of psychological well-being or competence." Traumatic events, by definition, were "expected to overwhelm."[10]

These assumptions left little room for doubt. When there was acute trauma, the best we could hope for was suffering and then gradual recovery, much like the gradual emergence of healthy adjustment after extreme deprivation.[11] Indeed, when describing the best possible outcomes after potentially traumatic events, experts in the 1980s and 1990s often used the phrase "resilience as recovery." To some extent they still do today.[12]

If it were truly the case that acute trauma inevitably caused acute suffering, as almost everyone seemed to assume, then why even bother looking for resilience after people experienced potentially traumatic events? Researchers who studied these kinds of events, whether in children or adults, for the most part didn't bother. Their focus remained almost exclusively on the long-term costs. Probably for this reason more than any other, the first evidence for resilience following potentially traumatic events didn't come from the study of such events per se. Rather, it came from research on grief and loss. Actually, it came from my own research on grief and loss.

Patterns of Grief

I began to study bereavement in the early 1990s as a postdoctoral research fellow at the University of California, San Francisco. At that time, the dominant ideas on grieving were remarkably similar to the dominant ideas about trauma. Everything and everyone, it seemed, was focused on psychopathology. Just as trauma theorists had come to expect PTSD, bereavement experts nearly unanimously assumed that the death of a loved one inevitably resulted in prolonged suffering and grief. And like trauma theorists, bereavement experts thought the best possible outcome was one of a gradual but nonetheless still dreadfully painful recovery.

I was new to bereavement. How I got there is a longer story I've told in a previous book, *The Other Side of Sadness*.[13] But I was deeply skeptical. How could such a pessimistic scenario be true? Losing a loved one is undeniably painful, and it goes without saying that some bereaved people will be devastated for a long period. But the idea that most people would be shattered by the death of a loved one made no sense. How would the human race have survived this long?

Even more perplexing, at that time there was hardly any solid research on the broader reactions to bereavement. Almost everything that had been done had focused only on bereaved people who had been struggling for years. Concentrating so exclusively on prolonged grief reactions told us almost nothing about what grief was like for other people, including those who may have adjusted more quickly. And if we didn't understand how people coped effectively with loss, how could we hope to understand the extremes of suffering?

I had only just begun to study bereavement. I was young and unknown and my opinion didn't have much impact. But a few other, more well-known psychologists had already begun to voice similar concerns.[14]

I decided it was time to put these questions to the test. The first study my colleagues and I conducted took several years to complete. But the results squarely contradicted the traditional view of loss. It was obvious right away that many of our bereaved subjects were resilient. Some suffered from prolonged symptoms—consistently high levels of grief and depression across the first several years of bereavement. Also, not surprisingly, others experienced a more varied, gradual recovery pattern. But an impressively larger portion of the bereavement participants we had tracked showed almost no grief or depression, not even in the first few months of bereavement, and they continued to exhibit this healthy course for the remainder of the study.

This was not the "resilience as recovery" pattern that had been described by developmental psychologists. This was straight-up resilience, clear and simple. Of course, there was pain and sadness. Of course, there was some struggle. There is always suffering when someone important to us dies. But the resilient bereaved subjects seemed to be able to manage that pain and to continue meeting the ongoing challenges of their daily lives, even relatively early on. We saw it when we interviewed them. We saw it in their physiological responses, in their facial expressions, and in how they managed their emotional reactions.

Because resilience to grief was a new idea, we wanted to be extra sure we had it right. For example, we arranged for some of the participants to be evaluated independently by expert grief therapists in their own private offices, using whatever format they would normally use to assess a new patient. The expert therapists had no access to our data and knew nothing about our findings. Yet their assessments agreed with our own, again revealing clear evidence of resilience.[15]

At first, many bereavement experts were skeptical, and some of our colleagues dismissed our findings as a mere fluke. But as I continued on with this research, sometimes using different approaches, the same patterns emerged—chronic symptoms, gradual recovery, and resilience—only even more clearly.[16]

Eventually, I moved on to a faculty position at Columbia University's Teachers College in New York City. Although I continued my research on bereavement, my long-standing interest in trauma reactions also began to resurface. Earlier in my career, as part of my PhD training, I had completed a yearlong clinical placement working with military veterans who suffered from PTSD. During that rotation, I noticed that some of these veterans didn't actually appear to be suffering from PTSD even though they had been diagnosed with it. I wasn't sure what to make of this at the time. Since it was still early in my training, I simply stored the information away, somewhere in the back of my mind, and moved on. But in New York, almost a decade later, I began to think back to those nascent observations. I had by this point documented abundant resilience among bereaved people. Would I find the same pattern if I looked at more overtly trauma-inducing events, such as natural disasters or violent assaults? I had a very strong hunch that I would.

But where to begin? I had published some research on different kinds of potential trauma, but only in collaboration with other investigators. I needed my own data. But where would I find it? Where would I find trauma? As I was pondering this question, trauma found me.

When the World Collapses

The 9/11 terrorist attacks sent shock waves across the globe. Just about everybody expected the worst. The sheer magnitude of the attacks, coupled with the dramatic images and stories dominating the media, led to predictions of unprecedented levels of PTSD. New York City's health commissioner anticipated a looming "public mental health crisis." Crisis hotlines began to prepare for the inevitable "deluge" of calls they knew had to come. City officials consulted with trauma experts from around the country and "began making preparations to train an army of volunteer therapists." Not that the city wasn't already well prepared. As the *New York Times* observed, the city had "more psychotherapists and mental health agencies per square mile than anywhere in the country. Internationally known trauma experts taught at local universities. City officials, schooled by the 1993 bombing of the World Trade Center and the crash of Flight 800, were able to mobilize quickly and think creatively in a time of enormous turmoil." Still, even these officials wondered how they would manage to care for "a traumatized community" and meet "the needs that were sure to appear."[17]

An article in the popular magazine *Scientific American*, published soon after the attacks, predicted a surge in anxiety-related disorders across the country, especially for those directly affected in New York.[18] The kind of harrowing trauma so many New Yorkers had just lived through, it was assumed, would place extraordinary numbers in the highest-risk group for PTSD. Indeed, because "the emotional force of the attacks" was so powerful, "many officials suspected that even people used to coping on their own might seek professional help."[19] The Federal Emergency Management Agency (FEMA) must have thought so too. In the aftermath of the attacks, FEMA allocated an unprecedented surge of mental health aid, totaling hundreds of millions of dollars, to New York City to provide free crisis counseling to any and all comers.

One of the reasons expectations for enduring PTSD were so high was that the attacks involved exceptionally brutal and deliberate violence. As one trauma expert put it, "If an airplane had accidentally flown off course in a heavy fog in New York and taken down one of the towers, it would have been very traumatic but probably less traumatic than knowing that somebody, or some group, wanted to kill everybody in those buildings."[20] Of course, as the day unfolded, people directly affected came face to face with the stark realization that the horrific violence they had fled was no accident. It was a deliberate and shockingly callous act of terrorism. Against such a grim backdrop, it was difficult to imagine how anyone could *not* develop PTSD.

But was just about everyone close to the attack doomed to suffer? Was PTSD an inevitability? For most mental health professionals at the time, the answer was a resounding yes. Even those who were more cautious thought the probability of PTSD to be extremely high.

A Few PTSD Symptoms

The earliest research seemed to confirm these dire predictions. Within only three days of the attacks, the RAND Survey Research Group began polling a representative sample of people from across the United States.[21] Their findings made headlines. Forty-four percent, close to half of those surveyed, reported one or more symptoms of extreme stress. For those within a hundred miles of New York City, the proportion was even higher, 61 percent of their sample. The researchers at RAND are well respected for their methodological rigor, and they were appropriately cautious about making too much of their initial results. They noted, for example, that most trauma studies report only the prevalence of disorders and not symptom counts. Without comparison data for symptom counts, it was difficult to know what having one or more symptoms of extreme stress actually meant. Nonetheless, they still had enough confidence in their findings to conclude at the end of the report that "the psychological effects of the recent terrorist attacks are unlikely to disappear soon."

It wasn't long before other data began to appear that seemed to confirm the RAND findings. Among the most carefully conducted studies were those by Sandro Galea and his colleagues at the New York Academy of Medicine. They focused only on New York, surveying Manhattan residents from five to eight weeks after the attacks. Because New York is an extremely diverse city, ethnically and culturally, they were especially careful to survey a representative sample of the population. Their initial results echoed the RAND study. Most Manhattan residents, around 58 percent, were suffering from one or more PTSD symptoms.[22]

A few PTSD symptoms are one thing. What about actual instances of the disorder? Here the story was more nuanced. A much smaller proportion, only around 7.5 percent of Manhattan residents, had met criteria for PTSD. The proportion was higher for those living south of Canal Street, close to the World Trade Center site. In this case, the prevalence of PTSD rose to 20 percent. And when the researchers examined data from people who were directly affected by the attack—for example, people who were in the World Trade Center when the planes struck—the PTSD prevalence rose higher still, to close to 30 percent.[23]

These were weighty numbers. Only a little more than a month after September 11, already close to one in three people directly affected by the attacks were reporting symptoms strong enough to qualify as full-blown PTSD. It seemed an ominous confirmation of the direst predictions.

Yet these early PTSD numbers could also be taken to show the opposite. Many survivors did not have PTSD. In fact, the majority of those who had endured direct exposure to what was turning out to be the most devastating terrorist attack on record in the United States had not yet developed PTSD. It was still early, however, and many observers expected that the PTSD numbers would continue to rise.

And then, to just about everyone's surprise, the rates precipitously dropped. When Galea's team studied the situation again six months after the attack, they found that the prevalence of PTSD among Manhattan residents had shrunk from the initial prevalence of 7.5 percent to less than 1 percent.[24] The PTSD rates were still higher among those directly affected by the attacks, but these numbers, too, had declined. The change was so pronounced that Galea and his colleagues concluded that there had been "a rapid resolution of most of the probable PTSD symptoms in the general population of New York City."[25]

The same story—the surprising lack of evidence for enduring trauma—was also witnessed in the use—or more accurately, the lack of use—of crisis counseling in the aftermath of the attacks. The millions that FEMA had provided for New York City to offer free crisis counseling appeared to have been misguided. Simply put, almost nobody seemed to want it. Even in the early days after the attacks, the volunteers manning psychiatric emergency rooms and clinics found they had little to do. People were not using these services.[26]

At first it was assumed that it must have been due to stigma. People were not coming for counseling because they felt it was a sign of weakness. Or perhaps they were afraid to face their trauma, or simply didn't know the services were available. Ads were plastered in subways and on buildings publicizing the free treatments and encouraging any and all who might be interested to seek them out. Still they did not come. Well-meaning but frustrated counselors began looking for customers themselves, sometimes cold-calling companies affected by the attacks to offer their services. In some cases, volunteer counselors wandered into firehouses or snuck past the barricades at ground zero to see if the rescue workers might be interested. Although such a forceful approach may have been welcome for some particularly distraught survivors, pressuring people into treatment can and often does backfire. In the end, this approach was likely to have done more harm than good.[27]

How do we make sense of this pattern? What did it mean that so many people early after the attacks had "one or more symptoms of PTSD"? This simple piece of data, and the response it evoked, shows strikingly how easily we become blind to the possibility of genuine psychological resilience. The phrase "symptoms of PTSD" sounds bad. But in actuality, the phrase has no practical or scientific meaning. "Symptoms of PTSD" could mean one symptom or just a few symptoms or many symptoms. Or it could mean nothing more than a few common, everyday problems.

Consider, as an analogy, a minor skin rash. A skin rash can be unpleasant. It can also be a sign of a number of serious medical problems, including several life-threatening diseases, such as toxic shock syndrome, Rocky Mountain spotted fever, and even cancer.[28] For this reason alone we should pay attention to skin rashes. But by the same token, we need to keep in mind that skin rashes are also commonplace, usually transient, and often indicate nothing more than a minor irritation or allergic reaction. By itself, in the absence of other symptoms, a skin rash is usually benign. It is only when it co-occurs with other critical indicators, such as fever, pain, swelling, nausea, headache, diarrhea, or vomiting, that there is any real cause for alarm.

The same is true for psychological symptoms. The RAND study reported that a large number of people had at least one symptom of extreme stress. The researchers came to this conclusion by asking their respondents about five symptoms: feeling irritable, having difficulty concentrating, having trouble falling or staying asleep, feeling upset at reminders of the attacks, and experiencing disturbing dreams and memories about the attacks. Only two of these symptoms directly referenced 9/11: feeling upset by reminders and experiencing disturbing dreams and memories. The possibility that large numbers of people might have reported these reactions so early on shouldn't have been at all surprising. The 9/11 attacks occurred on a Tuesday. The RAND survey began only three days later, on a Friday. At that point, the attacks were very much on everyone's mind. They dominated the newspapers, television, and the Internet. The Friday after the attacks, the first day of the survey, was also the first weekend, and a day that was designated by then president George W. Bush as a National Day of Mourning. Given this backdrop, or I should say despite this backdrop, the more interesting data to report would have been how many people were *not* feeling upset by reminders or dreaming about the attacks.

What about the remaining symptoms in the RAND survey: irritability, difficulty concentrating, and sleep problems? These are symptoms included in the PTSD diagnosis. But more important, they are also common woes. The RAND team had pointed out that there was almost no comparable data on symptom counts that they could use to make sense of their findings. That was certainly true at the time. Almost all the research available was on the presence or absence of the diagnosis; for people who were not diagnosed with PTSD, symptom counts were simply not recorded. A couple of years later, my research team and I decided that we needed to collect data on these same symptoms, so that we could examine just how common such symptoms might actually be. Our results showed that most of what the 9/11 surveys were tapping into, when they reported that so many people had at least some PTSD symptoms, was in fact probably the normal emotional backdrop of daily life.

In one study, for example, we measured each of the symptoms of PTSD in a group of people who had not been exposed to any recent trauma. Not surprisingly, very few people in this group met the criteria for the PTSD diagnosis. The rate of PTSD was at the same low level reported in national surveys of non-exposed populations.[29] But when we examined the frequency of individual symptoms, we found a different story: around 40 percent of our subjects had at least one symptom from the PTSD diagnosis. In other words, even when there is no recent trauma and almost no PTSD, 40 percent of people in the general public are likely to report one or more of the same kinds of problems—irritability, trouble concentrating, sleep difficulties—observed in PTSD. This didn't mean they had some PTSD. To the contrary, when a few symptoms of PTSD occur in isolation, they are usually just responses to common everyday troubles.

The Resilience Blind Spot

On September 11, 2002, the one-year anniversary of the attack, the American Psychological Association published a short report with the title "What Have We Learned Since 9/11? Psychologists Share Their Thoughts on Lessons Learned and Where to Go from Here." Not all of the psychologists who contributed to the report were ready to accept that the early signs of trauma were misinterpreted, or that their predictions might have been misguided, or even that the widespread trauma everyone expected didn't happen. Ignoring this potentially embarrassing point, they focused instead on how the 9/11 attacks had revealed new ways we could be traumatized or new sources of anxiety that might plague us in the future. But the most poignant reflection, and the most honest, came from Patricia Resick, a renowned trauma researcher and director of the University of Missouri's Center for Trauma Recovery. She did not mince words: "People's expectations about the impact of the attack on the country's mental health were wrong," she wrote. "Lesson? Strong emotions do not equal psychopathology."[30]

It's difficult to overstate the significance of Resick's words. They point directly to what may be the biggest lesson from 9/11. Most people exposed to highly aversive or life-threatening events experience lingering short-term effects: a few days or even weeks of distress, troubled dreams or nightmares, a sense of dread when reminded about the event. These responses are perfectly natural. They indicate the fact that our stress response is hard at work trying to help us adapt. But short-term traumatic stress is not PTSD. Even a few weeks of traumatic stress is not PTSD. We only get into the realm of PTSD when that traumatic stress doesn't go away.[31]

The nature of these early, transient distress reactions seems to confuse us. They blind us to our own capacity for resilience. I call this failure *the resilience blind spot* because of its similarity to blind spots in our visual system. Each of us has a visual blind spot, only we don't notice it. What we see with our eyes is created by millions of photoreceptors layered over the retina at the back of the eyeball. These photoreceptors connect to other, intermediate neurons and are eventually gathered together to form the optic nerve, which exits through the retina and then travels to the brain to create visual perception. Because the spot on the retina where the optic nerve exits has no photoreceptors, unavoidably each eye has a blind spot. It's almost impossible for us to actually "see" the blind spot unless we close one eye and do a certain exercise. Even then, it's very difficult. That's because our brains estimate the information that should have been in that spot, and then fill it in so that we have a seamless perceptual experience.

Metaphorically, the resilience blind spot works the same way. Potentially traumatic events are almost always disturbing. They make us feel frightened and vulnerable, and they rivet our perceptions to visceral danger. We see nothing but threat, and find it hard to even imagine not suffering. Resilience, in that context, doesn't even enter the picture.

Our blind spot for resilience is often reinforced by pronunciations from the mental health world. Not that this should be particularly surprising. The mental health profession has grown steadily since World War II. Psychology, psychiatry, and social work were once thought of as odd and unusual professions. They are now among the most common and well respected. Psychological experts can be found in our schools, workplaces, universities, and government agencies. Over the years, we have come to rely on these experts to help us negotiate the seemingly endless challenges of the modern world. Psychological experts help us to study and to be more productive; they advise us on our eating habits, our substance use, our sleep, and our relationships; they warn us about technology; they reveal to us what makes us happy and what likely does not—and much more.

Owing to the rapid ascension of the idea of PTSD, psychological experts specializing in trauma have been awarded an especially prominent degree of authority. But our understanding—even our awareness—of our responses to potentially traumatic events is still new and still limited. Quite naturally, then, when such events occur, we turn to trauma experts for guidance. And because we have little else to rely on, when trauma specialists tell us "trauma is everywhere," we believe it.[32] When they say that trauma "runs through our individual lives and through our world," and that "no one is untouched by trauma," we believe that, too.[33] We believe them when they write of "the ubiquity of trauma," and when they describe trauma as "an indivisible part of human existence" that "takes many forms but spares no one."[34] And when something as ghastly as the 9/11 attacks happens, and trauma experts tell us we are headed for a mental health crisis, we have no choice but to believe that as well.

The question, though, is not why we so readily accept such dire predictions, but why, given the still limited understanding of trauma and PTSD, these predictions are made with such absolute confidence in the first place.

·

DR. JENNIFER DYCKMAN works in a mental health clinic in a large midwestern suburb (she is an amalgam of actual therapists I have met, but I have altered key details to conceal both her identity and that of the clinic). The clinic is an active place. In addition to providing individual and group psychotherapy, it regularly offers educational events and training workshops for therapists in the surrounding community.

Dr. Dyckman is a founding member of the clinic and a specialist in psychological trauma. She's been a therapist for well over twenty years and at the clinic for the past thirteen. On a typical day she will see up to four individual patients, participate in one or two group therapy sessions, sit in on organizational meetings, and work individually with the junior therapists whom she supervises. It's a busy schedule, but Dr. Dyckman loves the work. She rarely finds it boring or tiring.

Like most of her colleagues, she tries to keep up with the professional literature. She reads the journals and attends professional conferences. But she has found that, over the years, the new research has held less and less interest for her. The professional meetings have become for her more a way to network with colleagues than to learn about new ideas. Most of the research articles she reads seem irrelevant, with little practical use for her day-to-day work with patients. This doesn't bother Dr. Dyckman. She is confident in her abilities, and she is widely acknowledged in the clinic as one of its leaders. She knows trauma inside and out, and when a traumatized patient walks through the clinic doors, she feels she will do as good a job as anyone in caring for that patient. By all accounts, she has the right to be confident. She is very good at what she does.

But there is a flip side. Therapists like Dr. Dyckman rarely see people during the course of their work who have been exposed to potentially traumatic events and remained symptom free. That's because people who do *not* develop PTSD symptoms have no particular reason to seek out a mental health professional. And because trauma therapists like Dr. Dyckman usually do not see people who might be resilient to trauma, they tend to think resilience is much less common than it actually is. In other words, they tend to develop their own resilience blind spot.

Why is this a problem? If Dr. Dyckman is good at treating PTSD, why should she care? What difference does it make if she is estimating the prevalence of resilience accurately as long as she is helping the patients who really need help? Actually, there would be no problem at all, as long as only severely traumatized patients walked through the clinic doors. The complications only begin when there is ambiguity. When it's not clear whether someone is suffering from PTSD, then a resilience blind spot becomes more of an issue.

In the ambiguous cases, traumatic stress might be misdiagnosed as PTSD, for example. Or, worse, problems that emerge independent of a trauma reaction—problems such as loneliness, fatigue, or depression—might be viewed as just another variant of PTSD and treated as such. Similarly problematic, sometimes potentially traumatic events, such as the 9/11 attacks, change a person's life in a way that is confusing or disorienting, or just plain difficult, but not necessarily traumatic. These problems, too, can easily be misattributed to PTSD. And when that happens, whatever intervention might be considered would be targeting the wrong problem.

The even more pernicious problem, though, is that this kind of blind spot leads us to doubt that resilience can ever be genuine. We become suspicious. Where there is genuine recovery, we see deception. Where there is strength, we see weakness. Where there is optimism, we see only denial—and a dark future filled with hidden trauma symptoms lurking just below the surface. Insidiously, the resilience blind spot can lead us to doubt our natural abilities. It can do this so thoroughly, in fact, that a team of therapists once published a paper dismissing resilience as the "illusion of mental health."[35]

Shortcuts and Distributions

As striking as this kind of dissonance may be, it is nonetheless also perfectly understandable. Therapists are not unintelligent. All licensed psychotherapists in the United States must have an advanced degree from an accredited training institution. No, the source of the resilience blind spot has very little to do with intelligence or training. Instead, it stems from a simple set of very human mistakes to which almost everybody—therapists and laypeople alike—are susceptible.

Two psychologists, Amos Tversky and Daniel Kahneman, devoted their careers to studying these kinds of mistakes. Their research has been enormously influential. For Daniel Kahneman, it led to a Nobel Prize (Amos Tversky died several years before the prize was awarded, and sadly, by the rules of the committee, his name could not be included). At the crux of their research lies a set of shortcuts they called "intuitive heuristics."[36] We use these heuristics, they showed, because of the immense amount of information we are confronted with during the course of a normal day. The average person makes thousands and thousands of quick, practical decisions every day, often with incomplete information. We rely on heuristic shortcuts to make sense of it all. Often, these shortcuts work pretty well. But they also frequently lead us in the wrong direction.

One of the more common shortcuts is the *representativeness heuristic*. We use this heuristic when we assume someone or something belongs to a certain category merely because that person or thing seems to match our stereotype for the category. We might assume a person is a college professor, for example, because he or she seems to dress and behave like our image of a college professor. But, as Tversky and Kahneman pointed out, the representativeness heuristic can cause people to make incorrect judgments.[37] In our example, college professor is not actually a very common occupation, so the heuristic could well mislead us.

Another shortcut is the *availability heuristic*. We use this heuristic when we decide how frequent or probable an event might be based on how easily we can bring examples of that event to mind. In other words, we are biased by how *available* the examples are, and we mistake availability for actual frequency. A poignant illustration of the availability heuristic comes from the fear of flying. Many people are uneasy flying. It's not a completely irrational fear, because airplanes do occasionally crash, and when they do, the consequences are usually dismal. But airplane crashes also make for dramatic and disturbing images that are hard to forget, especially when we are on an airplane and there is a sudden burst of turbulence. If there has been a recent crash in the news, we might succumb to another common heuristic error, called *anchoring*. In this case, we anchor our judgments based on the most recent piece of information we have. In actuality, the probability of an airplane crash is extraordinarily low. Yes, airplanes do occasionally crash, but relative to the vast number of airplanes in the sky at any one moment, the rate is infinitesimal.

We are all susceptible to these mistakes. But what about highly trained professionals—doctors or lawyers, or, for that matter, mental health professionals? With all their training, wouldn't they be able to avoid these kinds of misjudgments? Somewhat surprisingly, the answer is no.[38] Psychotherapists have been found to rely especially heavily on heuristic shortcuts.[39]

Just how far off are heuristic-driven misjudgments about trauma and resilience? What does the actual distribution look like? Most readers of this book will have, in one way or another, heard about distributions. We are usually taught in school that when we take a lot of measurements on something—say people's heights—we tend to get a *normal distribution*. You may have also heard this described as a Gaussian distribution, or, in visual terms, as a *bell curve*. That's because normal distributions are shaped like a bell. Most of the measurements cluster pretty close to some midpoint, the statistical average, and then spread out in either direction like the flanges on a bell (left side of Figure 1). We get a normal distribution for height because most people are of relatively similar height, and thus will clump together in the middle, while relatively fewer people are at the extremes of tallness or shortness.

Conventional wisdom suggests that mental health should also be normally distributed. Most people are reasonably healthy, we assume, so they should clump in the middle of the distribution, and there should be relatively fewer people at the extremes of either poor mental health or exceptionally good mental health. But actually, this is not true. Mental health is usually not normally distributed. Typically, it produces what we call a "positively skewed distribution" (right side of Figure 1).

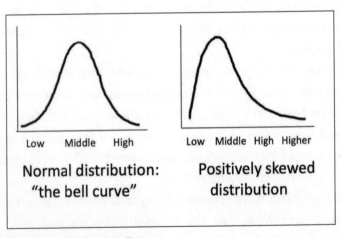

Normal distribution: "the bell curve"

Positively skewed distribution

FIGURE 1. Distribution Curves

Consider depression, for example. The number of people with symptoms of depression usually form an asymmetrical bell curve. The large number of people who have relatively low levels of depression symptoms form a large cluster close to the low end of the depression scale. There are relatively fewer people with high depression scores, and in this case the range extends pretty far up the scale along the positive end. As a result, we get a long tail that forms a positive skew shape.[40]

What happens to the distribution of scores for mental health when there is a potentially traumatic event? Conventional wisdom in this case suggests that, since most people are deeply affected by potentially traumatic events, the entire distribution of symptoms will simply slide up toward higher symptom scores. But this assumption also turns out to be wrong. In the aftermath of a potentially traumatic event, the distribution of symptom scores changes only slightly—it flattens out some and tends to extend farther up the scale—but most people are still clustered pretty much near the bottom of the scale. In fact, this is true regardless of whether we are talking about symptoms of depression, of grief, or of PTSD.

To my mind, this is simple but strong evidence for human resilience. You can see the pattern clearly in the graphs shown in Figure 2, where I've reproduced the actual distributions of symptoms following several different types of potential traumas. These graphs represent the distributions in terms of frequency proportions at discrete levels of symptoms. These particular graphs come from studies we've done on different kinds of real-life events, including loss, traumatic injuries, and a mass shooting, based on different kinds of symptoms—PTSD, grief, depression, and general distress. As far as potential trauma goes, these are all unquestionably severe challenges. Yet, in each graph, the clustering of symptom scores at the low end is obvious. In other words, without anything more sophisticated than a simple picture of the distribution, we can see that most people are resilient.

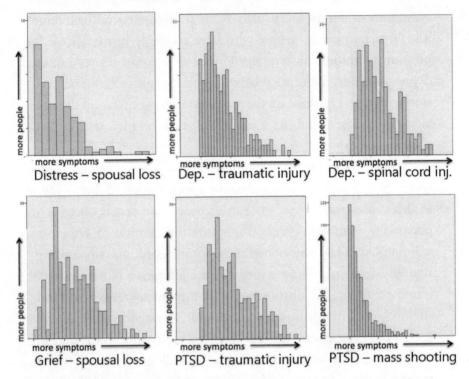

FIGURE 2. Symptom Distribution Following Potential Traumas

Graphs were created using data from the following studies: T. A. DeRoon-Cassini, A. D. Mancini, M. D. Rusch, and G. A. Bonanno, "Psychopathology and Resilience Following Traumatic Injury: A Latent Growth Mixture Model Analysis," *Rehabilitation Psychology* 55, no. 1 (2010): 1–11; G. A. Bonanno, C. B. Wortman, D. R. Lehman, R. G. Tweed, M. Haring, J. Sonnega, D. Carr, and R. M. Nesse, "Resilience to Loss and Chronic Grief: A Prospective Study from Preloss to 18-Months Postloss," *Journal of Personality and Social Psychology* 83, no. 5 (2002): 1150–1164; I. R. Galatzer-Levy and G. A. Bonanno, "Optimism and Death: Predicting the Course and Consequences of Depression Trajectories in Response to Heart Attack," *Psychological Science* 24, no. 12 (2014): 2177–2188; G. A. Bonanno, P. Kennedy, I. Galatzer-Levy, P. Lude, and M. L. Elfström, "Trajectories of Resilience, Depression, and Anxiety Following Spinal Cord Injury," *Rehabilitation Psychology* 57, no. 3 (2012): 236–247; H. K. Orcutt, G. A. Bonanno, S. M. Hannan, and L. R. Miron, "Prospective Trajectories of Posttraumatic Stress in College Women Following a Campus Mass Shooting," *Journal of Traumatic Stress* 2, no. 3 (2014): 249–256.

The graphs tell us something else. If you look closely, you can see that they do not form perfectly smooth curves. Actually, they are not curved at all. They are jagged and bumpy. Those bumps, it turns out, are enormously important. It means that the distribution is probably multimodal, or, more plainly, that people are clustering together at different spots in the distribution. Each graph is a little bit different. But generally, it looks like those at the low-symptom end of the scale, the people I describe as resilient, tend to cluster into one group. It also looks like there may be a few other groups—one or two in the middle, for example, and maybe one higher up the scale. If I had created similar graphs at different points in time, we would see similar groupings. But crucially, we would also see that some of the groups had shifted around within the distribution. This gives us another important clue. It means that the groupings of people in the distribution are changing over time. In other words, they are forming trajectories.

The Resilience Trajectory

When the September 11 attack on the World Trade Center began, I was uptown, literally miles away, in my office at Columbia University. My wife emailed me shortly afterward to say that a plane had struck Tower 1, the North Tower. Like just about everybody else, I pictured a small private airplane. A tragic mistake by a confused pilot. Almost certainly people had died. Two or three, maybe more. I didn't think much more about it.

A bit later, I ventured out into the hallway. There I was surprised to find that a number of my colleagues had gathered into small clusters. They were speaking in hushed tones. Their fright was palpable. Everyone seemed to know that something of greater magnitude was unfolding, but what exactly was not yet clear.

I walked over to the tallest building on campus on the chance that I might be able to see the towers. The building was already in the process of being evacuated and the elevator had been locked, but the stairway was still accessible. I decided to walk up and take a quick look. As I climbed the stairs, I passed several colleagues making their way down. They walked in hurried silence. One colleague looked at me and simply shook his head, as if to say, "What a terrible thing." I picked up my pace, reached the top flight of stairs, and walked out onto the roof.

The sight brought me to my knees.

I could see the towers clearly. The North Tower was billowing smoke. An enormous gray-black cloud was filling the sky and drifting eastward.

Like so many people that day, I watched in stunned silence, transfixed, unable to move.

I don't remember how long I remained on the roof. A few minutes? A half hour?

At some point, I ran back down the stairs and out to find my son at his preschool. The teachers were waiting for parents to arrive. I took his hand and we went quickly to a nearby park, where I knew I would find my wife and daughter.

Once we were all safely at home, I did what so many other New Yorkers did. I tried to make myself useful. I went as far downtown as I could. I volunteered. My colleagues and I organized a public forum. We made sure our clinic would stay open around the clock, in case anyone needed help.

After a few days passed, it became increasingly obvious that I had to find a way to learn from this event. The 9/11 attacks were tragic and distressing, but they were also unprecedented, and they gave us a chance to discover the full range of human reactions to such a large-scale trauma. I still wanted to study resilience, according to my original plan. But at that point, I wasn't sure whether that would be possible. It didn't matter. My goal now was to learn from the attacks in any way I could.

My research team got right down to it. We contacted as many people who had directly experienced the attacks as we could manage. We interviewed them and measured their behavior, their facial expressions, and their physiological responses. We conducted elaborate mental health assessments and then repeated these assessments several times over the next two years. Later, I collaborated with Sandro Galea, the epidemiologist I mentioned earlier who systematically collected data on the entire city.

We learned a great deal from these studies, including the fact that survivors showed the same three trajectories I had seen in my earlier research: chronic symptoms, gradual recovery, and resilience. I had seen these trajectories with grieving people, and now I had seen them unmistakably in people exposed to a large-scale terrorist attack. It was becoming clearer that these trajectories were likely prototypical responses that people would show when confronted with nearly any type of potential trauma. Above all, the resilience trajectory was again the most common of these prototypical responses. This finding helped me clarify my definition. The resilience trajectory is in evidence, I proposed, *when people in otherwise normal circumstances are exposed to an isolated and potentially highly disruptive event, but nonetheless maintain "a stable trajectory of healthy functioning across time"* (see Figure 3). [41]

Over the ensuing two decades, my research team and I continued to find evidence of these same trajectory responses. Along the way, other researchers also began mapping trajectories, and the evidence gradually piled up. Isaac Galatzer-Levy, my student Sandy Huang, and I tallied up the results of sixty-seven different trajectory analyses in 2018. The results were remarkably consistent: in almost every analysis, the resilience trajectory was the most common pattern observed. [42]

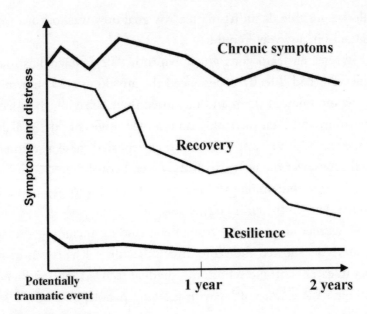

FIGURE 3. Resilience Trajectory over Time

Adapted from Bonanno (2004).

Sometimes, the prevalence was quite high. For example, soldiers who were assessed before they deployed for combat operations and then repeatedly in the years afterward showed impressively high resilience. I was involved in one such study that used data from a massive project called the Millennium Cohort Study. This study was a *prospective study*, meaning that it followed the soldiers from before to after their military deployment. In fact, it was the largest population-based prospective study in US military history, involving well over one hundred thousand US soldiers.[43] When we plotted trajectories of PTSD symptoms from these data, we saw the resilience trajectory—a pattern of little or no PTSD symptoms—in 83 percent of the soldiers.[44] This prevalence was unusually high. Why? There are several possible reasons, but the most likely had to do with the fact that soldiers are exhaustively trained prior to deployment. The more we know about a potentially traumatic experience—what is likely to happen, how it will unfold over time, and so on—the better equipped we will be to handle it.

But this level of preparation is unusual. Civilians who experience traumatic injuries—for example, from car crashes, serious accidents, or gunshot wounds—usually have no warning and no chance for preparation. A typical day for someone who suffers this kind of injury begins the same way any other day begins, except at some point that person finds himself or herself in an ambulance speeding on the way to the trauma unit of the nearest hospital. Not surprisingly, given the frightening nature of such events, many of the people who go through them show a chronic trajectory of elevated PTSD symptoms. Nonetheless, the resilience trajectory still consistently emerges as the most prevalent outcome, ranging from 62 to 73 percent across the studies.[45]

We've also seen the resilience trajectory at roughly this same prevalence in studies of other severe events, such as natural disasters, sexual and physical assaults, and even mass shootings. The prevalence was again similar following acute, life-threatening medical events, such as finding out that one has cancer, or experiencing a heart attack.[46] And we've continued to see the resilience trajectory at more or less this same frequency in people who have experienced the death of a loved one, and also, more recently, in people who have suffered other types of losses, such as divorce or the loss of a job.[47] Across all of these different studies, the resilience trajectory was always the most common outcome, occurring, on average, in about two-thirds of participants. In other words, a healthy majority. A healthy two-thirds majority.

New Questions

The striking prevalence of resilience across so many different types of possible trauma slowly but surely shifted the paradigm. New questions began to emerge. Instead of asking only about what goes wrong, about what falls apart after traumatic stress, it was now possible to ask about what goes right. It was possible to probe that resilient majority—that two-thirds—to find out how they were managing it, to learn what it was they were doing that allowed them to adapt so well. But this wasn't just a shift from bad to good outcomes. It didn't mean we could now ignore more severe trauma reactions. To the contrary, the inclusion of resilience in the picture only broadened the view. It meant that, as we learned more about what people showing resilience were doing, we could also begin to understand how that knowledge might be used to help other people, the one-third or so who were suffering more extreme reactions.

The only problem was that insights into what resilient people were actually doing, at least initially, turned out to be surprisingly elusive.

PART II

Stories and Predictions

CHAPTER 3

More Than Meets the Eye

A fter Jed emerged from the coma, he took stock of all that had happened. He had been crushed by a twenty-five-ton sanitation truck. His body had been rearranged and his left leg was gone. It was easily the worst thing that had ever happened to him. Yet, remarkably, he had only a fleeting trauma reaction and no lasting trauma symptoms. We've now seen that resilience is actually the most common response to potential trauma, and against that backdrop Jed's fortitude begins to seem less surprising. Maybe if he had known about these results, he too would have been less surprised.

But, surprised or not, we still need answers. We still need to know wny Jed coped so well. How did it come about? Was it something in him? Or something he did? One way to gain some insight is to look more closely at his experiences. Perhaps then we might see some indicators, something he said or the way he managed himself during the accident, that might have foretold his salubrious outcome.

There was one brief but compelling moment on the night of the accident, at the hospital. Just before he was taken into surgery, Jed seemed to rise above the terror. Although he was already losing consciousness and fading in and out, he recalled how the arrival of his girlfriend, Megan, had bolstered him. He was optimistic. He remembered feeling "really confident" as they wheeled him off to surgery, almost as if he already knew on some level that he was "going to be okay." Optimism and confidence are not insignificant sentiments, and we'll explore them further later in the book. But for now, we have this small sign. Does it tell us anything? And, if so, what?

Conventional wisdom about trauma would no doubt dismiss the possibility out of hand. This was one brief instance. Weighed against the entirety of what was otherwise an overwhelmingly brutal experience, how could such a fleeting moment actually have had much impact? The resilience blind spot would of course influence this judgment. But beyond that caveat, skeptics could also point out that more severe or "traumatic" experiences have, in fact, consistently been shown to produce more severe and extreme trauma outcomes, not resilience.[1] We know, for example, that disasters involving mass violence tend to produce greater psychological impairment, and less resilience, than technological disasters, which in turn tend to be more harmful than natural disasters.[2] We also saw a clear influence of severity of exposure on the prevalence of resilience in our 9/11 research. People who reported being physically injured in the attack, for example, had the lowest levels of resilience of anyone in our study.[3]

If the impact of trauma severity is as clear as these findings suggest, then we are still left with no explanation for Jed's seemingly instantaneous return to psychological equilibrium. There was also the burden of his having been in a coma for so long. What little we do know about medically induced comas does not appear to lend them any obvious psychological benefits. To the contrary, as we saw, they often manufacture traumatic memories of their own. Again, though, Jed seemed to have brushed these memories away, too, and with equal alacrity.

What about accounts from other people who had endured severe and potentially traumatic events? If we explored these accounts, perhaps then we'd see more straightforward signs of either enduring trauma or resilience. First-person reports of extreme traumatic stress as vivid and detailed as Jed's are not easy to come by. Fortuitously, though, as part of our 9/11 research, we routinely conducted extensive interviews with survivors. Three of those interviews were particularly compelling. Each of the interviews was with someone who was in the World Trade Center when the attacks had occurred. Each interviewee had endured what seemed like an endless onslaught of overwhelming fright, terror, and confusion. Each one barely escaped the collapse of the buildings. Their personal accounts of that day provided us with rare glimpses into what is typically an unreachable and inaccessible aspect of human experience. For that reason alone, their stories are worth exploring further. But these accounts do not just tell us a great deal about the hidden world of potential trauma; they also give us a perfect opportunity to consider the questions at hand. If someone is likely to experience prolonged trauma or PTSD, for example, would we see it early on, in that person's account of the experience? And what of resilience? Might the things people say or do at this early juncture serve as a harbinger of a more salubrious outcome?

Will, Reina, and Eva

Eva had just started working at the World Trade Center in Tower 2, the South Tower. She was settling into her desk in an office about halfway up the tower when, sometime after 8:30 a.m., she heard the explosion. She wasn't sure what it was. One hears noises from time to time in tall buildings. You shrug and you go back to whatever you were doing. But Eva could tell right away that this noise was different.

Will heard it too. He had just exited the subway and was making his way through the crowded main transit concourse below the World Trade Center. At that time of day, the concourse is already in full throttle. Streams of people intersecting, swerving, somehow just missing each other.

And then, BOOM.

Commuters bumped and turned and looked to each other. Will could see the concern on their faces. He felt anxious. He remembered thinking something like, "You don't hear a noise like that in a building this large unless something bad just happened."

Reina was much closer to the impact, as she worked on one of the upper floors of the North Tower. She had just walked out of her office and into the corridor when a thunderous explosion startled her. She let out a spastic whimper. At first, she was embarrassed. Then just frightened.

"I ran down the hall to where some of my coworkers were standing," she said. "Everyone was looking around, and looking at each other, with this confused expression on their faces. They were all talking at once."

Reina couldn't decipher it. Someone yelled for calm. Someone else shouted out directions. Another yelled to move to the middle of the office. Someone said something about a bomb.

And then, abruptly, all eyes riveted to the scene unfolding outside the windows.

"You could see fireballs," Reina told us. "We had these enormous windows. Orange and black and smoke and fire, above us. Fireballs, whooshing out, from above, toward the South Tower. From somewhere above. Like someone had one of those things in the movies, a fireball machine, you know, a giant weapon . . . a flame thrower, like something in a movie."

•

AT FIRST, EVA didn't realize the danger she was in. She and several coworkers had gathered around the window to see if they could tell where the sounds came from. The day was so beautiful, the sky so incredibly clear and blue, it was hard to believe anything could possibly be wrong. Except for the paper. Streamers of office paper, blown out by the explosion above, had begun to flutter down across their windows. To Eva it looked like a ticker tape parade.

One of Eva's coworkers decided they should evacuate. Eva pondered this. There had been no announcements. No alarms. But clearly something was wrong with the building. She decided it might be best to leave and made her way to the stairwell.

But where was it?

Eva searched for the stairwell but couldn't find it. She felt disoriented, and then she realized that she had lost track of her coworkers. She began to panic. She saw some people going through a door at the end of the hall. She followed. To her relief it led to a stairway, and she hurriedly began her way down. Almost immediately her progress slowed. The stairwell was already crowded. There were a lot of people below her, and she could see people coming down from the flights above. In those few brief moments, Eva realized that she was in serious danger and no one around her was familiar. She felt alone and frightened and began to cry.

·

HIGH ABOVE, IN the North Tower, Reina was already struggling to survive, and she hadn't yet left her office.

The floors above her had just absorbed the impact of a jumbo jet. The building shuddered and then began to sway. "It was really strong," she later said. "I thought, 'Oh my God, the whole building is going to topple over, and we are just going to slide into the South Tower.' It was all happening so fast. My mind was racing. It was terrifying, because, you know. I mean, we were so high up."

Reina grabbed onto a desk. She wasn't sure why, and she remembers thinking that it didn't really make sense. If the tower fell, a desk wouldn't help her. But she needed to hold on to something. Anything.

People began to shout and run toward the stairs. Reina abandoned the desk and followed. She turned down a corridor. There, she was confronted with an incomprehensible sight. The office was completely destroyed. What moments ago was an orderly array of pristine white walls and wood paneled doors was now a blackened mess. Wood and wires hung indiscriminately. Oddly shaped pieces of metal jutted out. People had bits of ceiling in their hair and on their suits; blood and dirt stained their faces. Through a doorway, Reina saw fire.

She felt her heart pounding in her chest.

A crowd was trying to enter the stairway. Reina told herself to be calm. She tried not to push, but her mind was screaming. She shuffled along, and when she finally reached the steps, she was ready to run.

"I was not thinking much. I was on automatic pilot. But I was pretty scared, and I was taking the steps, you know, fast. I was like running down the steps. I am in pretty good shape. I wanted to go. . . . I wanted out of there. I knew it was a long way down. That was somewhere in the back of my mind. I don't think I had any idea about how hard it would be. I was just like, 'Let's get the hell out of here . . . as fast as I can.'"

Reina's progress inevitably slowed as the stairwell became more crowded. She fought off panic: "It occurred to me that with all these people, so many people, the stairwell could clog. And it was getting hot, really hot. Then we'd be trapped."

It took Reina a long time afterward to piece together how long she'd been in that stairwell. For most of the descent, she had little sense of where she was in the building, or for that matter, what had actually happened. The heat was unbearable. The air grew heavy and stale and was everywhere permeated by a strong chemical smell, maybe gasoline. Reina's eyes stung. She used the collar of her blouse to try to shield her face. There was glass in the stairwell and then water. And then more water. The water began to puddle up. It became more difficult to negotiate the debris. But she kept going.

Most unforgettable were the images of the people she encountered on the way down. There were those who tried to push their way ahead, to save themselves first. But most people took the steps in grim silence. Some seemed to be in shock. Others were undoubtedly overwhelmed by fear. Some people were in pretty bad shape. Women in business heels, for example, found it impossible to negotiate the rubble that had gathered in the stairwell. They had no choice but to remove their shoes and go barefoot through the glass, metal, and seeping water. Reina thanked the heavens that she had decided to wear comfortable shoes that morning.

At several points, she encountered small clusters of people who had been badly burned. The experience was as incomprehensible as it was unnerving. "Everyone made way for them. Let them pass," she recalled. "They looked really awful. I saw someone's skin was gooey, like she was covered with paste. Their cloths were torn. Just bits of clothing, hanging on them, like a . . . I had never seen anyone burned. I didn't know what it looked like. I was not sure what I was seeing. I still remember one woman's face. She was badly burned and she just kind of stared, blank."

A bit later, Reina crossed paths with a group of firefighters who were making their way up the tower. These images still haunt her.

"These guys with all this heavy equipment. The stairwell was so hot, and they were lumbering their way up. They were calm, like soldiers, you know, going into battle. I remember how calm their faces looked. This was their job. They do this kind of stuff. They were a comforting sight, but I know they're all dead now, you know. I mean they must be. They would have to all be dead now. All of them. They were going up. They wouldn't have made it. Nobody knew the tower was going to come down. They were going up to fix it."

•

As Eva and Reina struggled with their descent, Will was making his way through his own version of the catastrophe. Confusion had spread through the transit concourse. Will lingered for a short while, to see if he could learn more about what had happened, and then decided it was best to leave. Oddly, he found himself disoriented, unsure of where he was. The exit he would have normally taken was blocked. People were running about and then everything suddenly looked different. Will's memory of what exactly happened next is fuzzy. Either he couldn't remember or he couldn't find the alternative routes out of the building. He grew anxious and confused and at some point realized he was going in circles. Then finally, after what seemed like a very long time, he found a passage to street level.

As Will emerged into daylight, he was surprised to find himself in the middle of a disaster scene. Crowds of onlookers had gathered. Police were everywhere and several areas had already been cordoned off.

He struggled to comprehend the unfolding scene outside. His confusion and uncertainty gave way gradually at first and then in large chunks to the dawning terror of the event. He noticed almost immediately that many in the crowd were staring upward and pointing. There was a great deal of smoke, but he couldn't see much else. As he struggled to get a better view, his mind grabbed bits and pieces of conversation. Not much of it made any sense.

He walked on and then looked up again. Now he could see it clearly. A cavernous hole in the tower, too large to be possible, and flames, and an enormous plume of smoke rising and drifting eastward. How could this be? The sheer incomprehensibility of it all stopped Will in his tracks. He had no idea what to do next. He just stared for what seemed like a very long time. He was dumbfounded.

At some point, Will came to his senses long enough to realize that he was still in danger. Parts of the building were falling off, and many people around him looked badly shaken. He was thinking that he should move farther away when suddenly people in the crowd began to scream. Will looked up. He could see that something else from the building had just fallen. Every part of his body wanted to bolt, but he couldn't make himself move. He couldn't help but study the object as it fell. He had never seen anything fall from so high up. It was a relatively small piece, but still obviously dangerous. Will then noticed that it was moving. And it had smaller parts that were moving. To his horror he realized he was looking at human arms. This was not a piece of the building. This was a human being.

Why? Will couldn't make any sense of it. Logic had already been inverted by the events of the day, and now someone was plunging through the sky to a sudden death. Why? Why would anyone be falling from so high up? Why at that moment? Had the person been thrown by the blast? What was happening up there?

It was not until much later, when Will actually had time to think and had more of the facts, that he was able to piece it together. People who worked on the uppermost floors of the North Tower, above where the plane hit, had been trapped. There was no way down past the flames, and tragically, no means of rescuing them from above. When the plane hit, it exploded into a gigantic ball of flames. The building began to roast and crumble. For those trapped above, the heat quickly became unbearable. They gathered at the open windows and gasped for air. And finally, when it was clear there was no way out, someone simply flung himself into the clear blue sky and plunged to his death. Then others followed. Most likely their hearts gave out before they reached the ground, more than one hundred stories below. All the crowd could do was watch in abject horror. With each jump, they screamed and then fell into spooky silence, and then screamed again.

Will could not process it.

"I can't explain it. I never felt anything like that in my life. Never. Never. Never. Never saw anything like that. Never in my life."

•

EVA WAS NOT as high up as Reina, so she made it to the bottom of the stairwell sooner. But she still knew little about what had happened. She was exhausted and frightened, but she thought at least her ordeal was finally over. She would walk out into the trade center plaza where there were stores and people and that would be the end of it. Only that's not what happened. The stairwell exited in a location, still inside the building, that Eva was not familiar with. She had no idea where she was. After roaming about in confusion for some time, she finally spotted a familiar landmark and made her way to a set of glass doors that led to the plaza. That exit was now blocked, but through the glass Eva got a glimpse of the devastation that was in progress. The plaza was covered in ash. There were fires, and objects were falling, and then Eva, too, heard the crowd scream in horror.

She jerked her head away. She couldn't see farther up the towers and she didn't yet know what had happened to cause these appalling scenes. The illogical nature of it all stunned and disoriented her, and she went into a kind of numb shock. Then she simply wandered off, unsure of where she was going. Somehow, she found herself on a moving escalator. She heard a man speaking loudly on a cell phone. She heard him say an airplane had hit Tower 1, the North Tower. That news was just as illogical. She couldn't put it together. How could it be?

She wandered farther, still somewhere inside, her mind drifting in a way that later, with hindsight, seemed to her completely nonsensical. She noticed that all the stores were closed. Normally, at that time of day, the stores would be open and bustling with activity. Why were they closed? She saw a small group of people gathered at a corner where two television monitors were broadcasting. She walked up to them.

That's when she snapped out of it.

"I guess the monitors were for watching the stocks. And it was there I saw a live shot on CNN of Tower 1. It was the first time I saw it. There were a few of us. I don't know how many, a few people standing around, like idiots. And, and I'm watching the TV, and that's when I kind of woke up. I was like, 'Oh my God.' It was so horrible. What a horrible thing."

Eva's body woke up, too. She made her way as fast as she could toward the subway. A Port Authority guard told her the entrance was blocked and led her to an exit onto Liberty Street. She reached the street for the first time and then walked out into the unfolding chaos.

The streets were already blanketed with ash. People were standing about looking upward. Eva no longer remembers what happened next, but somehow she ended up next to Trinity Church, directly in front of the South Tower. She was looking up when suddenly, directly above her, the second plane slammed into the tower.

"It was the most horrible thing I've ever seen. It was like, I don't know, I'm looking up and I see this massive white tube going right into the building. It was very fast. What was it? I had no idea. A missile? A huge missile? A whole bunch of things happened very quickly. I remember thinking, 'What caused this?' I was trying to put it all together. It wasn't a separate incident. How did that happen? I think this was the first time that I had that feeling of being in a war. Alarms were going off in me."

People were running and screaming. Eva turned to run, but then a large man ran past her. They collided. He pushed her out of the way. His forearm struck her, and she went down. She was stupefied.

"This was the first time I felt like I was going to die. I thought I was going to get trampled. I thought they were going to knock me to the ground, and they were just gonna run right over me. Even now, I think about how miraculous it was that nothing hit me. The fact that this huge airplane hit this huge building, and nothing hit me, is unbelievable."

Eva picked herself up, gulped air, and ran. She didn't know what to do or where to go. She just ran.

•

By the time Reina finally reached the bottom of the stairs, planes had struck both towers. The descent had exhausted her. She had walked down more than eighty flights of stairs under excruciating conditions. Like Eva, as she exited the stairwell she expected that the worst part of her ordeal would be over, and like Eva she was surprised by the chaos and destruction in the plaza. Unlike Eva, though, Reina did not learn about the reason for that chaos and destruction until she finally made her way out to street level.

"When I walked out, I was so relieved. It was bright out. The sun was, you know, there was this intense blue sky and it was very bright. I was out. It was . . . such a wave of relief."

Her thoughts turned immediately to her family. She was sure they were worried. She planned to call her husband and her children's school to let them know she was okay. But her relief just as quickly faded as she was overwhelmed by a circus of people and police and vehicles. She struggled to get through the crowd, to move away from the trade center to where she could gather her wits.

And then she looked back, up at the towers.

"I don't even know how to say, how to explain, I mean how it felt. I am not sure . . . it was just, like, 'Wow. What?' The towers were in flames, and there was dark smoke. Just an enormous amount of smoke. So much. Dark, and these orange flames. Both towers. Huge clouds of smoke, like you know just pouring out."

The crowd took on a new meaning. Now she saw the fear and panic in their faces. She peppered anyone nearby with hurried questions. How could this happen? What is going on? She learned about the planes. She learned that the Pentagon in Washington had also been hit. And she heard that it all seemed to be part of a major terrorist assault. She studied the towers again.

"And that was, I guess . . . and it was then I realized . . . this is it. This is . . . I don't know what, really, and I thought, 'This is coming down! These towers are coming down. And they are going to crush me.'"

Reina's exhaustion vanished. She ran as fast as she could.

•

WILL WAS TRYING to pull himself together. The sight of human bodies falling from the North Tower stunned him. Something had gone terribly wrong, and he knew that he'd better get himself out of there. But as horrific as the sight was, he couldn't tear himself away. He began to walk backward. Then he walked sideways, still looking back, and then he finally forced himself to turn away. He broke into a run. He was no longer sure where he was. He ran for several blocks, confused, and once he felt he had gone a safer distance, he sat down. He didn't know what else to do.

It was then that he heard a strange, deep sound, like metal groaning. He could feel it. One of the towers was literally breaking up inside.

He saw large chunks of the building coming down. Then an even larger piece broke off. Will knew what it meant. He stood up, but he couldn't move. He just stood there watching. He was transfixed, frozen. He could see the building begin to sag. He could hear it. The building was collapsing.

"I was still watching. Standing there, watching. And then the ground started to rumble. People started screaming and running. Screaming. I finally realized, 'This is it. It's going to come down, and it's going to kill me.' And I ran."

All was chaos. Will ran past broken windows. He saw a group of people huddled in an entryway. He squeezed in with them. Other people ran by. His entire body was twitching. He thought he should keep running but he couldn't move again. The rumble grew louder and louder and soon it was deafening. One by one, the people who had been huddled in with Will bolted back out into the street. Will leaned forward and looked up into the canyon of buildings. Then, he saw it.

"There it was. A huge avalanche, like a rumbling monster. Smoke. Dust. A gigantic dark cloud. It was . . . I don't know. It didn't seem real. It was racing up through this corridor of buildings, billowing. Incredibly fast. It was rushing right toward us. And then my brain or my mind or . . . I just ran. I mean I just ran, and as fast as I could. And I thought, 'This is it.' I really thought, 'I am going to die.'"

He didn't get very far. The rumbling cloud overtook him, flung him to the ground, and swept him up into darkness. He could barely see. He heard footsteps but he couldn't make anything out. He pulled his shirt up to cover his face and stumbled forward. He collided with people. He ricocheted off walls, objects, cars. The world was disappearing in an envelope of dust and ash. Will hit his head on something. It was another person. He heard a voice and then he lost his balance and slid to the pavement. He was swimming in ash. He told himself, "Get up. Just keep going. You have to get away from this." And he got up and he stumbled, and he ran.

He saw what looked like a door, half open. He made a split-second decision to enter. That decision just may have saved his life. The world quieted. Will coughed and tried to catch his breath. There was a light, but he couldn't see. His face and eyes were filled with dust and dirt. He was retching.

Will gradually made out that he was in a large room, maybe the lobby of a building. He couldn't tell. There were other people in the room. They were talking excitedly. Someone said they had to leave. The building wasn't safe. There was yelling. People were arguing. Will could hardly hear or see. His heart was pounding, and he was still coughing. He began to catch his breath, and then he made another spit-second decision. He turned and ran back out into the street.

Will had no idea how long he had been in the building. It seemed like only a few seconds, but once he was back outside, the dust cloud had lessened.

"I was still terrified, you know, but I began to think a bit more clearly. I thought maybe I can get to the river. I didn't know where I was. I couldn't make anything out. But I thought I had been going east. If I was, then eventually, you know, I would come to the East River. Alarms were still going off in my head, the panic button, and I thought, 'I can swim to Brooklyn. I can float. I can swim.'"

.

MEANWHILE, REINA WAS beginning to panic. She ran up Fulton Street but found it glutted with people. She pushed her way through anyway and then caught a glimpse of the Brooklyn Bridge between two buildings. Her mind was racing.

"I thought, 'I should take the bridge. I'll get out of there, across the river.' But then I was confused. I stopped and I was standing, and all this stuff was moving, all around me. I was . . . I thought, maybe the bridge wasn't such a good idea. It would be a target, for sure. I was like a wind-up motor. I was moving in different directions. You know, like I was a wind-up toy. I kept changing my mind. I ran uptown, north I guess, up Nassau. Maybe it was William Street? I don't remember now. I looped back . . . and then I changed my mind again and ran toward the entrance to the bridge."

Reina made it to City Hall Park and then her progress ground to a halt. The scene was mayhem. A crowd of onlookers had filled the park. Loudspeakers blared to "evacuate the area." Fire trucks honked, slowly edging forward, trying to get through. Police were having a difficult time of it. The crowd did not move. Some people were crying. Others were taking photos. Someone was filming.

Reina paused to look back at the World Trade Center.

"This was the first chance I had to get a good look. I saw the flames and smoke, and I had just been there! I was trying to make sense, you know, of that. I thought, 'How . . . ?', you know, I couldn't take it in. I was trying to collect my thoughts. Maybe make a phone call. And I wanted to take a good look.

"It was the most unbelievable sight. I mean, it just didn't seem possible. It wasn't . . . it was unreal. I told myself I would only stop . . . Not long. It was insane to stop. I mean it's a terrorist attack. City Hall would be a target, right? Government buildings. But I had to, to watch. It felt safer, you know, around, with other people, even though it wasn't really. It wasn't a smart thing. My mind was racing. I think I was kind of running in place."

An older man gave Reina a faint smile and held out a bottle of water. His kindness touched her. She drank a bit and handed it back. He motioned to keep it. She poured some of it over her head. More people turned to her. They began to ask questions. Reina realized that she looked a mess. She was disheveled and covered in dust and dirt. People began talking rapidly. Reina couldn't hear what they were saying and stepped out into the street to get a better view. It was then that she saw and felt what Will was seeing and feeling just a few streets over.

"There was this god-awful rumble, and one of the towers just shook and started collapsing," Reina said. "The North, er . . . the South Tower. It just imploded. You know, that was when . . . it just started collapsing in on itself and coming down. The most frightening thing I'd ever seen. I mean, all this huge building, and concrete and steel and glass. This gigantic building crumbling, and people, and it was . . . I began to cry, I remember that, and then I bolted. It was coming down so fast. I ran like I had springs in my feet. To this day, I am not exactly sure, I don't even know if I would have been caught up in it, but I just ran. I didn't wait to find out."

.

WILL WAS RUNNING, too. He found himself somewhere between the Brooklyn Bridge and the Manhattan Bridge and decided it was best to get off the island. The Manhattan Bridge was probably a better idea, he reasoned, but the Brooklyn Bridge was closer. He jogged over and joined the masses of people going up the ramp.

It was as if he'd joined up with a ghost army. Many of those walking the bridge had been caught up in the same cloud that had engulfed him. Their faces and hair were coated in white, like the characters in a bad zombie movie.

The crowd moved slowly. Will felt edgy. He tried to push his way through. Someone gave him a look. Another person yelled at him. Will couldn't make it out. He didn't care and he didn't wait to find out. The idea of walking across the bridge made him intolerably anxious. By this point, he realized he was in the midst of a terrorist attack. Although he wasn't thinking very clearly, he knew the bridge could be a target. It was a mighty structure, but at that moment, it seemed like nothing more than a fragile span that could easily come down and plunge him into the East River. And he knew he was going to be stuck on the bridge for some time.

He noticed that quite a few people had stopped. They were looking back, toward Manhattan. Will pushed on. "What the hell is wrong with you people?" he asked out loud. The crowd was not co-operating. Will felt as if he were pushing against a human wall. Their faces were riveted, frozen in anguish. Then something else began to register, something more like shock or disbelief. Will turned around.

"This was the first time I saw what had happened. There was a huge cloud of smoke and no building. Only one tower was left, and the other . . . it was just gone. Just completely gone. I could hear my heart pounding in my ears. I turned and I kept going. I wanted more than ever to get off that bridge. Then some people began screaming. I turned and looked again, and then I saw the second tower, it was going down too. 'My god.' I didn't watch. Not this time. I turned and I just plowed into whoever was in my path. I was like, 'Get the hell out of my way.' I am out of here, man. Move aside."

•

EVA NEVER SAW the towers come down. She was spared that shock, but not much else. After witnessing what she thought was an incomprehensibly huge missile (the second plane) slam into the South Tower literally directly over her head, only minutes after she had exited it, and then feeling that she would be trampled by people fleeing the danger, she picked herself up and ran. She had no idea where she was going.

She hadn't gone very far when she spied a set of gilded revolving doors. She thought to herself, "I'm going in, I'm going in those doors." The doors weren't actually gilded, which Eva determined several months later when she retraced her steps. But they looked safe nonetheless and Eva ran inside.

"I don't remember hearing the explosion. I'm sure I heard it. I must have heard it. But the only thing I remember hearing were screams. People were screaming, everybody. I was not. I was too scared to scream. I couldn't. I was hardly breathing. I was so scared that I was taking these very shallow breaths."

The building Eva had gone into was a school. She had the thought that she wouldn't be allowed to stay, that a guard would appear and tell her she had to leave. But there was no guard in sight. She walked across the lobby to an elevator, leaned against the wall, and slid to the ground, collapsing into a fetal position.

After a few minutes Eva noticed another woman in the lobby who was sobbing uncontrollably. Someone else, a janitor perhaps, was comforting her. Eva found a strange solace in the scene. Then a few other people appeared. Eva got up and someone hurried them all into what looked like an auditorium.

None of them were sure what was actually happening. Eva did her best to piece together the hurried conversations. She still thought she had witnessed a large missile striking the South Tower, and she knew she was still close, only about half a block from the trade center. Fear gripped her. Periodically, other people, other survivors, would enter the auditorium. Each time the door opened, smoke poured in and someone in the group yelled, "Close the door, it's a fire door. Keep it closed."

Eventually someone decided—Eva has no idea who—that everyone in the auditorium should be evacuated to nearby Battery Park. Eva had paired up with the woman who had been sobbing in the lobby, who was calmer now. The two talked and decided they would refuse to go.

"We were so adamant. It's very odd to remember, but we were, like, in commando mode. You know, we were thinking, 'Where are we going to be safe? Where are they not going to see us?' Right, and we felt that Battery Park was too open; they could drop things on us from the sky."

But then, to Eva's surprise, a group of children appeared. They shuffled into the room in single file, holding hands. Eva wasn't sure where they came from, but their appearance comforted her. Someone instructed her to follow along behind with the children. Not knowing what else to do, she complied. And together, they filed back out into the mayhem.

"We got out onto the street. Everyone was running. And then—I must have heard the sound. I don't, I don't remember. But I saw that the building—the South Tower—had come down. I had no idea that the building fell until I saw it was gone. I had no idea. But, oh my God, that was horrible. That was the worst part of the day."

As they neared the park, Eva and the woman she had paired up with reiterated their refusal.

"We said we didn't want to go in. It was a bad idea. Then the police finally came and said, 'Look. Please. We need you to go into the park.' You couldn't see anything. You couldn't breathe. Everybody was running. I didn't know what was happening. I expected people with machine guns to come out of the smoke and shoot. I really and truly believed that that's what was going to happen. People were just screaming and running, and it was just, it was horrible."

Eva's fear overwhelmed her. She tried to hide by leaning herself against a building. She remembers thinking that somehow if she could make herself look like part of the building, camouflage herself, she would be safer, less of a target. The other woman gave her a crazy look, took her arm, and motioned for her to follow. Eva did.

"It had become so dark. And I didn't know where I was. I mean, we were walking in darkness. I had no idea where anyone was. I couldn't see more than a few feet. And then, finally, the smoke started to clear and there was the blue sky again. I forgot. I had forgotten that the sun was out, and I was actually happy. It was crazy, I know, but I felt suddenly happy. I tried to put my sunglasses on but they were covered in soot, everything was covered in soot. And it was all over the streets. And people had, like, you know, just big piles of it on their shoulders."

Eva and her companion discussed whether they should attempt to get onto the Brooklyn Bridge. As they talked, a well-appointed man in a business suit and carrying a suitcase appeared out of nowhere. He had overheard their conversation. He told them he was from out of town and had only planned to be in Manhattan for the day. Eva found his presence calming, almost comical. "It was like *The Wizard of Oz*. You know, we said, 'Why don't you just come with us?'" Soon an elderly woman approached them, and they invited her to join them as well.

The group, now four people, made their way to the Brooklyn Bridge, but they were fearful. Like Will, Eva felt apprehensive about the bridge. It was too much of a landmark, and she thought it would be a target. They walked a bit farther and then decided the Manhattan Bridge would be a safer bet. Still, Eva found it "very, very scary."

She did the best she could to contain her anxiety as they traversed the bridge, but she struggled with one recurring thought: "I couldn't understand why some guy would try to kill me. Some guy tried to kill me, some guy I don't even know. I just, I didn't understand how that could happen."

Finally, after what seemed like an eternity, they descended the steps off the bridge and onto Jay Street in Brooklyn. To Eva's amazement, there they found a waiting city bus, "just sitting there." They got on and they were immediately peppered with questions.

"I told them where we just came from. This was the first time we were with people that weren't there, which was odd because, up until that point, everyone we saw was affected by it directly. And all of a sudden, it's like, we were in a new place and people were like, 'Oh my God.' You know, everybody knew. It was probably 11:30 a.m. Everyone by this time knew what was going on, what happened. Everything was closing up. And I thought, 'Maybe this is over. Maybe this god-awful experience is finally over.'"

Bringing It Home

Back when we conducted these interviews, our goal was to be as objective and professional as possible. Even so, listening to stories like these, so soon after the attacks, often had us on the edge of our seats. But as gripping as they may be, we still have our question: Based on the details of each account, can we predict who struggled more or for longer afterward, and who was resilient?

Some of you reading along may have already formulated your own hypotheses. Some of you may have even correctly matched the outcomes with the person. I am sorry to say, though, that if you did, it was probably a lucky guess. I've conducted this same exercise, informally, with different groups of people. Each time, I ask them to read these same accounts and then predict the outcome. The results overall have always been more or less random. This is no slight toward you, or toward anybody. It's just a very difficult task. There's so much going on in these accounts, it's easy to imagine just about any outcome. There are clues in each narrative that would seem to predict an enduring trauma reaction. But there are also plenty of signs of engagement and effective coping. So much so that it seems equally plausible that all three might have shown a resilient trajectory.

In truth, each person showed a unique outcome. Will suffered the most and for the longest. He struggled for several years with nearly debilitating PTSD symptoms that typified the *chronic trajectory*. Eva also suffered in the aftermath of September 11 and, for a time, everything for her was extremely difficult. But her struggle over the ensuing year followed a more manageable course typical of a gradual *recovery trajectory*. Reina showed the best outcome. She had some traumatic stress early on, but it didn't last very long. Her course clearly followed a *resilience trajectory*.

What if I had told you earlier, before you read the narratives, that each of the three exemplified one of these trajectories? Would the additional information have helped? In fact, it would have, because you would have at least known the probabilities. You'd have known that, since each person showed one of the three possible outcomes, even if you guessed randomly you would still have at least a 33.3 percent chance of hitting the mark.

I tried this version of the exercise on a group of people. I explained the three outcomes—chronic, recovery, and resilience—and told them that each person showed one of these outcomes, and each one was different. It didn't matter. The results were more or less random. The task was still too difficult.

What if I asked trained clinicians? Would clinical expertise make any difference? We've already seen that clinical judgments can easily go astray as a result of heuristic biases, and there is also the resilience blind spot to consider. With that in mind, we might suppose that clinicians might assume that none of the accounts could have led to resilience. But then again, if they knew that one of the three had shown a resilient outcome, this information should, to some extent, neutralize the resilience blind spot, allowing them to better utilize their clinical expertise.

When I tried this exercise informally with a group of practicing clinicians, most of them found the task quite difficult. And many were completely off in their predictions. But a good number were not, and as a group the clinicians were able to match Reina to the resilience trajectory at a level greater than chance. But only barely. They picked Reina as the resilient person only about 45 percent of the time. Given that random guessing would have yielded 33 percent accuracy, 45 percent is actually a pretty weak hit rate. Looking at it from another angle, we could say that even though they knew that one of the three people was resilient, more often than not—55 percent of the time—the clinicians still failed to identify that person.

Okay, then how do we square this up with the research findings? Why are clinical judgments, at least those based on written transcripts, so poor compared to the research indicating that trauma severity predicts a worse trauma outcome? Actually, they aren't. When we take a closer look at the statistical relationship in the research studies, we find that it, too, is surprisingly modest.

This is a good time to pause, briefly, to consider what a statistical relationship actually means. Trauma severity and trauma outcome are correlated. But when two things are correlated at a rate greater than chance, this tells us only that when one happens, the other is also likely to happen. It doesn't mean they always co-occur, or even that they necessarily co-occur most of the time. Violent crime, for example, tends to increase at higher temperatures, but we wouldn't take that to mean that if we go outdoors on a hot day we are going to be mugged. The correlation is not nearly that strong. The same goes for trauma severity and trauma outcome. They correlate only weakly, which means that trauma severity co-occurs with more extreme trauma outcomes only a relatively small fraction of the time.

Take, for example, the large population-based study of military combat deployment I mentioned in the previous chapter. If you recall, an unusually large proportion of soldiers in that study, 83 percent, had shown a resilience trajectory. When we looked at the impact of combat exposure, we found that soldiers with the most severe levels of combat exposure—things like witnessing maimed solders or civilians—were statistically less likely to show a resilience trajectory. Thus, severe combat exposure makes it harder to be resilient. Yet, compared to the overall prevalence of resilience in the study, the difference was actually quite small. The vast majority of soldiers with severe combat exposure, 81 percent, still showed a resilience trajectory.[4] This is not an isolated story. Other studies have reported similarly weak severity effects, and in some studies, the effects of trauma severity were dramatically reduced or even erased when other factors were taken into consideration.[5]

When we put all this together, it seems pretty clear that although trauma severity is broadly related to trauma outcome, that relationship is far from the whole story. There is clearly a lot more to it, and whatever that "more" might be should tell us something important about how resilience works. But actually, the implications go much deeper even than that. Trauma severity is the tip of the iceberg. When we expand our lens to other traits and behaviors that correlate with resilience, we get a bit of a surprise. Actually, we get a paradox.

CHAPTER 4

The Resilience Paradox

In the first few weeks after coming to, Jed's condition stabilized. He began to ponder his future. The course of his life had been radically altered. He was still so weak he could barely sit up. But he knew that eventually he was going to have to learn how to live in the world with a quarter of his body missing. It would be demanding and at times discouraging. And what of his girlfriend, Megan? Their budding romance had evolved into a long series of anxious hospital visits. It was, as Jed put it, "not what she signed on for." Would he have a normal sex life? Would their relationship survive? What about the fundamental milestones? Marriage? Children? Were these now out of reach?

A daunting reality loomed. Jed knew there would have to be a lengthy period of rehabilitation. He would have to learn to strengthen his upper body so that he could handle crutches or otherwise compensate for the absence of his leg. Then came the crushing news that there would be additional surgeries. Jed's medical team had labored intensively to save his life. But some of the procedures had only been temporary—stopgap efforts to keep him alive. Once he regained some of his strength, the surgeries would continue. That would mean more pain. As dire as it all sounded, Jed knew it was the best-case scenario, and it could yet be worse still. Medical procedures after major accidents are often unpredictable. There could be unforeseen complications and draining physical setbacks.

With these new tribulations on his mind, Jed began to feel the brunt of his loss. Although he never fell into a full-blown depression, he confided in me that he had nonetheless visited "some pretty dark places" and had sometimes struggled to find a way out.

His thoughts drifted back to the hospital bed, when he had first emerged from the coma. At that time, he had been flooded with anxious trauma memories. Then, the symptoms abated, remarkably quickly, in just a few days. Everyone was surprised, including Jed. He had no idea why the symptoms vanished. At first, he was puzzled, even curiously interested. Now, as the weight of this new round of challenges began to seep in, he felt an almost desperate quest for answers. Why was he so resilient the first time around? What was effective and what wasn't? He needed to know so that he could better equip himself for the struggles that almost inevitably lay ahead.

•

THE QUESTION OF what differentiates resilience from other, more severe responses to potential trauma has been staring me in the face for most of my career. When I first began looking for resilience, now three decades ago, my intent was solely to document its existence. Given the general consensus at the time that resilience was rare following potential trauma, I had to make sure I was right. But soon enough my colleagues and I had plenty of evidence that this was not an unusual story. Resilience was the norm. Only, like Jed when he emerged from the coma, we had precious few clues as to why. Years later, as the evidence piled up and we could see that the average prevalence rate for the resilience trajectory was around the two-thirds mark, the question became even more compelling. Why two-thirds?

And why, if most trauma-exposed people were able to find their way to stable health, was there always a sizable minority—on average around one-third—that continued to struggle?

We've seen already that trauma severity plays at least some role, albeit a surprisingly small one, in recovery, and that, obviously, there has to be more to it. Over the years my team and I have identified a number of behaviors and traits that correlate with resilience. Other researchers eventually joined in the hunt as well, and the list grew. News about resilience to trauma began to spread beyond the margins of academic research into popular books and media. More behaviors and traits were touted as resilience-promoting. Sometimes these popular works put forward the same characteristics researchers had identified, and sometimes not. And at some point, I am not exactly sure when, the list grew so large as to become more or less useless.

If we put it all together, listing every trait and behavior that has in one way or another been associated with resilience, whether in popular books and media or in academic journals, we get something like this: Resilient people are in control of their feelings, self-aware, and mindful. They pay attention to their bodily sensations. They're tolerant of painful emotions, acknowledge grief, and are able to face their own fears. They practice self-care, self-nurturance, self-compassion, and self-respect. They are curious, and they have a good sense of humor as well as a clear capacity for joy. They are optimistic, hopeful, and patient, but also tenacious and gritty. They have good problem-solving skills, set reasonable goals, take an action-oriented approach, and believe in their own abilities. They have a broad perspective, visualize resilience in their lives, and have the capacity to embrace change. When bad things happen, they write about them, find meaning, and identify as survivors rather than victims. They are able to transform adversity into opportunity. They are spiritual and religious, morally strong, practice thankfulness, and take time for solitude. They are involved in their lives, committed, and enjoy a sense of purpose. They have a clear sense of autonomy and control over their lives, but they are also altruistic, accepting, forgiving, and nonjudgmental. They recognize their own limitations and admit their mistakes, and they help others, but are also able to ask for help when they need it. They are securely attached to their closest family members and friends, and they have supportive relationships with many other people. They have good genes and they exercise regularly.[1]

Quite a list. All of these characteristics are undeniably good things to have or to be. But there are so many—who could have or be all of them? And more to the point, which ones would be the most likely to help us endure the extreme stress of potential trauma? Which ones would help us to be resilient to trauma?

Some of the characteristics certainly *seem* like they should promote resilience. Here's a prime example: religion and spirituality. Many popular lists include this factor. When I give public lectures on trauma and resilience, I inevitably get questions about religion and spirituality. It's not difficult to imagine why. Organized religion provides a stable belief system as well as affiliation and the shared support of a larger community. There is no shortage of anecdotes describing people who have found strength in their spiritual beliefs. Trauma therapists think so as well, proposing, for example, that the "personal quest for understanding" that characterizes a religious or spiritual focus "facilitates the integration of traumatic sensory fragments . . . thus working to decrease post-traumatic symptoms."[2]

So far so good. But is there any empirical evidence for such claims? One popular website assumed so when it unabashedly posted this emphatic headline: "Psychologists Have Found That a Spiritual Outlook Makes Humans More Resilient to Trauma."[3] The only problem is that the article that followed didn't actually discuss any evidence for that claim.

That's probably because there isn't any.

To be fair, spirituality is one of the more difficult concepts to measure. Although religious activities have been linked to good health in general, beyond that simple correlation things get complicated.[4] For one, our thoughts about God or religion are usually multifaceted, and in the context of life-threatening events, the way we think about these concepts often changes. When the chips are down, as the saying goes, some people find God. True enough, but some people can also experience more of a spiritual struggle: they may feel anger, or even a sense of betrayal, at the thought that God has abandoned them. Threat and conflict tend also to shift perceptions of God toward a more punitive deity.[5]

We could get around these problems, of course, if we knew for sure about a person's religion or spirituality before a potential trauma happened, and then tested whether it predicted resilience in the future, after the potential trauma. A prospective study of this nature is not easy to pull off, but it's not impossible. And actually, I was involved in a prospective bereavement study some years ago in which married individuals, several years prior to the death of their spouses, were asked how they felt about their religion of choice and whether they experienced a sense of a personal relationship with God. Positive answers to these questions correlate with good mental health. However, in our study they failed to predict a trajectory of resilience once participants were bereaved. In other words, neither people who felt positive about their personal religion nor people who felt a strong sense of connection with God were any more likely to be resilient several years later, after their spouses died, than other bereaved people in the study.

Here's another good example: mindfulness meditation. The practice of mindfulness meditation has become extremely popular over the past several decades and is a regular entry on many lists of resilience-promoting factors. Although it shares some similarities with religion and spirituality, in many ways it's an even more likely contender to actually promote resilience.[6] Like religion and spirituality, mindfulness can be measured using survey questionnaires, and it generally correlates with health and well-being.[7] But unlike spirituality, meditation can also be tested experimentally. We can't ask people to join a religion or develop spiritual beliefs for the sake of a psychology experiment. But we can invite them to participate in a ten-week mindfulness meditation course, and then compare their mental health to that of individuals in a non-meditating control group. Research using this kind of experimental approach has consistently shown mindfulness meditation to be genuinely effective in promoting health. It has, for example, been linked to improved mood, better job satisfaction, and even enhanced immune functioning.[8] When used as an intervention, meditation has also been shown to be effective for people suffering from serious psychological problems.[9]

Given such positive results, it's easy to assume that mindfulness meditation would help us manage the challenges of potential trauma. Full disclosure, I practice mindfulness meditation myself. I find it wonderfully useful in dealing with the stresses and strains of daily life. But personal experiences aside, science is science.

Unfortunately, there isn't actually any evidence that mindfulness predicts resilience.[10] Worse, there is at least some chance it could be detrimental. A group of mindfulness experts recently cautioned, in a paper published in a leading psychology journal, that misinformation about the effectiveness of mindfulness can mislead people, and can even lead to harm. An alarming number of published studies and case reports have linked meditation to serious side effects, including increased anxiety, panic, disorientation, hallucinations, and depersonalization—the feeling of being disconnected from oneself. It can also cause people who have gone through potentially traumatic events to reexperience memories of these events.[11] Reactions like these would be harmful under any circumstances, but they'd be especially damaging to people already made vulnerable by a recent experience of intense traumatic stress.

The Paradox

As disappointing as it may be that such seemingly healthy behaviors don't pan out, there are other characteristics that have been shown to have an empirical relationship to resilience. One of the best known is support from other people. Another is optimism, and relatedly, the belief in one's ability to cope well. People showing resilient outcomes also tend *not* to search for meaning after potential trauma, but rather to focus on problem solving. They are able to use a range of coping and emotion regulation strategies, and they frequently experience and express positive emotions such as happiness and joy. There are demographic correlates as well. For example, resilient outcomes are more common in people who are older, who have few additional stressors, and who have greater resources, such as higher income and education levels. And we have found that the different trajectories map onto distinct genetic profiles.[12]

These characteristics are meaningful and they give us plenty to work with in trying to understand how resilience comes about. But, unfortunately, we are not out of the woods yet. There is another snag. When we look closer at even these factors, we discover the same problem we saw with trauma severity. Although each of these characteristics shows a statistically demonstrable relationship to resilient outcomes, their actual influence on that outcome is surprisingly weak. Practically speaking, they tell us very little about who will likely show resilience and who will likely not. Even if we combine them—add them up—they still don't tell us much about the overall picture.

As mentioned earlier, I call this problem the resilience paradox. We know that a resilient outcome following potential trauma is common, and we know the characteristics that correlate with a resilient outcome, but, paradoxically, we still can't predict that resilient outcome with much accuracy. If you are not accustomed to this kind of talk about prediction accuracy, the idea probably sounds a bit odd. But in the world of inferential statistics it is well understood that many things in life influence us just a little bit.

It might help here to visualize a pie chart. Resilience after potential trauma is the pie. And when we try to predict resilience, we are essentially building the pie from individual slices of predictors. We have the trauma severity slice, the coping strategy slice, the social support slice, and so on. Now, because these pie slices have been empirically linked to resilient outcomes, it's natural to assume that they must be reasonably sized slices, and that once we put them all together, we'll have a nice full pie. I've depicted this version of the resilience pie on the left side of Figure 4. I call it the idealized resilience pie because it's the pie we assume we will end up with. Unfortunately, it's not a very realistic or accurate pie. The slices are actually pretty thin little slices, each accounting for a small portion of the pie. And when we put them all together, we tend to get something more like the pie on the right of Figure 4, the realistic resilience pie. You can see that we don't actually have a full pie. We don't have as much as half a pie.[13]

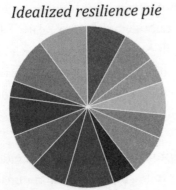
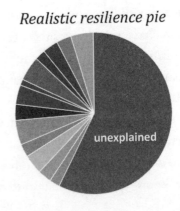

Idealized resilience pie   _Realistic resilience pie_

FIGURE 4. Resilience Pies

So how do we solve the resilience paradox? Maybe the solution has to do with the quality of the research. Typically, the predictors of resilience are measured by questionnaires. Maybe the questionnaires so far have simply been lousy questionnaires. Or maybe the research itself was flawed. We saw some of the problems that can plague research earlier, when we discussed studies on spirituality and mindfulness. These same concerns are definitely evident in at least some of the research on resilience. But it's not enough to explain the paradox. Even when we use only well-developed measures and rigorous research designs, we still find the same paradoxically small effects.[14]

There is a better solution. A compelling clue comes from a similar paradox identified in the 1960s by my late colleague at Columbia University Walter Mischel. Walter was well known for his research on the so-called marshmallow test, which led to new insights about delayed gratification, but his major contribution to psychology came from his work on personality.[15] One of the dominant ideas in psychology at the time, and to some extent still today, is that people have stable personality traits—that is, their behavior is consistent and predictable across situations. Walter and other researchers began to notice that correlations between personality traits and behavior are actually quite small. Even more troubling, when they measured behavior in multiple situations, they found surprisingly little consistency. Put differently, although people seem to have stable personality traits, their actual behavior is not consistent. This observation came to be known as the *personality paradox.*

Walter and his colleagues launched an ambitious research program on the personality paradox. In a typical study, they tracked people's behavior across different situations during the course of their normal daily lives. Then they categorized the situations into specific types. When they did this, they found that although people were not very consistent in their behavior across all situations, they did tend to be consistent in specific types of situations. For example, a person who is identified as extraverted on an extraversion questionnaire is not always extraverted. But that person will tend to be consistently extraverted in certain types of situations (even if not others). Walter and his colleagues called these patterns *situation-behavior profiles.*

If we extended this same logic to potentially traumatic events, then we could assume that resilience-linked behaviors have only small effects because people don't *always* engage in them: they exhibit the behaviors sometimes, or maybe a lot, but not necessarily in the new situations they are confronted with in the aftermath of a potential trauma. This is in fact the case, as we'll see shortly. But there is still more to it. There is still the question of why this would be the case. Why would people not always rely on a generally effective behavior like seeking support from others, or some other favorite coping strategy? The answer to that question takes us to the heart of the paradox. These behaviors are not always effective.

The stress induced by potentially traumatic events takes time to contend with, usually at least several days and often longer. In addition to the unwelcome cascade of distressing thoughts, memories, and emotions these events produce, they often create unique problems for us to solve, such as adjusting our normal routine, dealing with the loss of a home or job, or managing an injury. Sometimes, as was the case for Jed, they alter the course of our lives. It takes time to work all this out. Even the most resilient outcome typically involves at least some struggle. During that period, no one trait or behavior will always be effective. This is true of personality traits—for example, people are not extraverted in every situation because extraverted behavior is not appropriate in every situation—and it's true for the behaviors and traits that predict resilience. The demanding and enduring stress caused by potential trauma varies so greatly that no single behavior or trait could ever possibly be effective at every moment in that process. Indeed, if we broaden our scope further, we find that *no single behavior or trait is ever always effective.*

Pretty Peacocks and Speedy Cheetahs

Every behavior, every trait, has both benefits and costs. Depending on the situation, sometimes the benefits dominate, and sometimes the costs do. This is true literally everywhere in nature, from the largest mammals to even the smallest, single-celled creatures.[16] Take, for example, the stunningly beautiful tail of the peacock. Although I live in Manhattan, there are three peacocks in my neighborhood. They reside down the street from my apartment on the grounds of the famously unfinished Cathedral Church of Saint John the Divine. The cathedral grounds are large for Manhattan, covering several city blocks. The peacocks live in a small shelter near the back of the cathedral, but for the most part they have free rein. One day, as I walked past the cathedral, I chanced upon a wonderful spectacle. One of the peacocks had decided to leap up onto the stone wall that surrounds the cathedral grounds and unfurl his tail. Passing motorists were so taken by the sight that they literally stopped in their tracks, and in no time, they found themselves embroiled in a hopeless traffic jam.

Charles Darwin, the father of evolutionary theory, was obsessively interested in the peacock's tail. Darwin caused one of the biggest upheavals in the history of human thought when, in 1859, he published his landmark evolutionary treatise, *On the Origin of Species*.[17] Pretty much up until that point, the only going way to understand animal diversity was creationism, which held that all animals on earth, including humans, were divinely created in one fell swoop. Darwin argued, and demonstrated with years of carefully collected observations, that animal variation could be explained far better, and far more completely, as the product of a slow evolutionary process called natural selection. Animals responded to the survival demands of their habitats, he argued, by gradually evolving traits and behaviors that helped meet those demands. Over time, those traits and behaviors became characteristic of the species.

But the peacock's tail deeply troubled Darwin. A year after the publication of his famous book, he wrote that "the sight of a feather in a peacock's tail, whenever I gaze at it, makes me sick!"[18] The reason for such dramatic revulsion was that he couldn't explain it. Why would a large bird ever evolve such an attention-grabbing tail? As far as birds go, peacocks are huge and meaty—and therefore desirable as possible meals to hungry predators. They lose their tails each time they molt, but the tails grow back, and when they do, they command a great deal of attention. Predators in the vicinity would easily see them. The sheer size of a peacock's tail also severely impedes the peacock's ability to fly, which in turn limits the peacock's chance of escape. Together, these features render the peacock, if you'll pardon the pun, a sitting duck.

For Darwin and his nascent theory, the peacock was a conundrum. Traits that foster survival will tend to increase in the population and gradually shape a species' evolution. But a tail that impedes survival? How or why would such a tail ever have evolved?

Although it took him more than a decade, eventually Darwin found his solution.[19] In addition to the gradual evolution of traits through natural selection, he added a second mechanism, sexual selection. Having seen how the size and grandeur of the peacock's tail made it stand out, even in comparison with other colorful birds, Darwin reasoned that females "must, during a long line of descent, have appreciated this superiority; for they have unconsciously, by the continued preference of the most beautiful males, rendered the peacock the most splendid species of living bird."[20] Although he hadn't worked out all the details of sexual selection, and he didn't even yet know about genes, the intuition was remarkably astute. Traits that are attractive to potential mates increase the odds of reproduction, which, as researchers would later demonstrate, increases the odds that these traits will be passed on genetically.[21]

By expanding his view of species evolution to include these two competing mechanisms—natural selection for survival and sexual selection for reproduction—Darwin had beautifully demonstrated how the tension between costs and benefits can be literally built into an animal's nature. Large colorful tails increase the odds of reproduction, which is quite a bonus; but in situations where predators lurk, a large colorful tail makes it more likely that the animal will perish, which is not so good.

We see this same kind of cost and benefit trade-off in other creatures. For example, the cheetah. In this case, the tension is not sexual. It's about food. Cheetahs are marvelous specimens. They are sleek and remarkably fast—the fastest terrestrial mammals on the planet, able to accelerate to sixty miles per hour in only three seconds! They are also agile and, thanks to their lengthy tails, can turn on a dime. Their eyesight is excellent too, and, of course, they have teeth and claws. Put all these features together and it's hard to imagine a more perfectly evolved predator. When they are hungry, all they have to do, it would seem, is run down some food, eat their fill, and take a nap.

Although cheetahs do often spend most of their days lying around, their existence is not nearly so idyllic as it might seem. Their greatest asset—speed—is also their biggest liability. Because of the metabolic needs required for the level of speed cheetahs generate, they have relatively little stamina. They can only run for several hundred meters before they need to stop and rest. Tracking studies have shown that cheetahs end up abandoning most of their chases even when they are within striking range. They simply can't go on. And if they are lucky enough to quickly snag a meal, they are often so exhausted by the chase that they need to rest for up to thirty minutes before they can even eat it. By that time, other creatures are occasionally emboldened to sneak in and steal the kill.[22]

The Good, the Bad, and the Ugly

Humans are animals, too, and, not surprisingly, this same trade-off between costs and benefits applies to human behaviors. Consider coping and emotion regulation strategies. Numerous strategies have been identified, and it is commonly assumed that these strategies are either good or bad, either inherently useful and effective or else ineffective and possibly harmful. Extending this logic, it might naturally be assumed that healthy people almost always used the good strategies, the effective ones, while people who were struggling emotionally mostly engaged in the ineffective strategies.

One of the supposed good strategies, aptly named *problem-focused coping*, involves directly changing or modifying aspects of a situation that might be causing distress. Another presumed good strategy, known as *reappraisal*, involves changing the way we perceive a situation. We might, for example, feel angry when we encounter a particularly rude or hostile person, but then minimize our anger through reappraisal by reasoning that the person must be having a bad day.

An outright bad strategy, at least according to popular assumptions, is the intentional suppression of emotion. We engage in suppression when we try to force ourselves not to feel or show an emotional reaction. The presumption that suppression is ineffective probably had to do with observations that at times it can be difficult to pull off, especially when we are highly emotional. Suppression can also lead to interpersonal misunderstandings, as, for example, in social situations where people normally expect to see emotion.[23]

Early research seemed to confirm this basic good-bad taxonomy. But the evidence didn't hold up very well over time. First of all, although most people are pretty confident that they know which coping behaviors they use, what they actually do when coping is much more variable than they realize. In one persuasive study, for example, researchers first asked people how they typically coped with stressors, and then, over the next two days, probed them repeatedly about coping when they were actually going through stressors. Their original answers failed to predict what they actually did while coping in the moment. In another study, the same researchers reversed the procedure. They began with the two-day probing about actual coping behavior, and then, afterward, asked people to report on the strategies they had used over those two days. Again, there was little correspondence.[24]

The consequences of different strategies also show far more variability than a simple good-bad taxonomy would suggest. For example, although problem-focused coping has been found to be more effective than emotion-focused coping, in some types of stressor situations the opposite pattern has been observed.[25] Consider, also, the common assumption that expressing emotion is adaptive while suppressing it is harmful. Although there is research highlighting the costs of emotional suppression, overall the story is more or less equivocal. Actually, when the combined effect of over three hundred emotion regulation experiments was summarized using an approach known as meta-analysis, on balance emotional suppression proved moderately effective but, at the same time, varied depending on the type of event.[26]

That suppression would be useful in some situations only makes sense. It would be important, if not essential, for example, to conceal distress while engaged in public speaking, or to minimize the expression of anger while trying to resolve a conflict. The suppression of outward signs of emotion should also be beneficial, at least some of the time, in the context of extreme adversity. Although most people are willing to offer support to close friends or relatives when they look pained or upset, even if it means they might suffer themselves, over a long period of time emotional expression can frustrate and ultimately drive away otherwise well-meaning, supportive others.[27] Thus, it would be important to be able to minimize those expressions when the situation called for it. Anecdotally, I've heard this from many of the parents I've interviewed in my research on potential trauma. In times of emergency, they've told me, it is often necessary to mask their own distress to keep their children calm.

We even see variations in effectiveness for the reappraisal strategy. Although reappraisal is generally considered the most successful of all emotion regulation strategies, it is not always effective; in some situations, it can actually lead to worse outcomes. In the context of high life stress, for instance, reappraisal has been linked to lower depression, but only when the stress was uncontrollable. The researchers suggested that when a situation is uncontrollable, and thus there isn't much that can be done about it, the best course is to change one's emotions through reappraisal; but when the situation can be controlled, and thus something can be done about it, it's more effective to change the situation. It is in the latter context that reappraisal has been linked to increased depression. The same pattern is evident when people are tested on their preferred strategies in different situations that might involve reappraisal. Most people prefer to use reappraisal when they anticipate that a stressor will be relatively mild, and thus likely to be more controllable. For more extreme stressors, however, other strategies, such as distraction, are preferred more often.[28]

All of this research points to the same basic conclusion: coping and emotion regulation strategies are inherently neither good nor bad. Every strategy has costs and benefits, and a given strategy is effective only insofar as it helps us meet the demands of a specific situation. Ironically, this is not a new story. The leading theorists on coping and emotion regulation have always emphasized this kind of dynamic interaction with changing situational demands. The core theorists have also emphasized the importance of timing. What may be effective at the onset of a stressor event, they pointed out, may be less effective or less useful later as the stressor runs its course.[29]

The dynamic nature of regulatory processes stands out in even starker relief when we are confronted with traumatic stress. Extreme conditions oblige us to put aside our normal concerns and shift to what I have called *pragmatic coping*. We focus only on survival, on "whatever it takes" to get us through. And that "whatever it takes" can often involve strategies or behaviors that we wouldn't normally consider using, or, for that matter, that we normally wouldn't even consider healthy. For this reason, I've also referred to this kind of coping as *coping ugly*. When the chips are down, and we are struggling, whatever we do to get through it need not be pretty, or satisfy conventional wisdom. It just needs to work.[30]

Too Much of a Good Thing

There are some behaviors that seem so obviously beneficial that it's hard to imagine they would not always be helpful—for example, positive emotions. Although the benefits of positive emotions, such as joy, happiness, pride, and amusement, were more or less ignored in psychology for much of its history, they have received an enormous amount of attention in recent years and are now widely acknowledged as part and parcel of good mental health. How could they not be? Not only do positive emotions feel good, but there is an abundance of evidence linking them with a wide range of health benefits. The strength of this research has catapulted positive emotions into the limelight of public discourse and instigated a flurry of programs advocating their cultivation to foster optimal health and well-being.[31]

Once again, though, a closer look at the research dulls some of the luster. Like most things in life, positive emotions are beneficial primarily in moderation. Moderate levels of positive emotion can help us be more creative, for example, while extreme levels do not. Extreme positive emotions also lessen our awareness of danger and can interfere with our ability to inhibit risky behaviors. And, as is true for every human behavior, the usefulness of positive emotions depends on the situation. A case in point: positive emotions help us perform better when we need to cooperate with others, but they hinder our performance in situations that require some level of confrontation.

In competitive situations, expressing positive emotion can incur a serious social cost. In one research study, observers rated videos of people winning acting awards, sporting matches, and game shows. The winners who effusively expressed positive emotion were viewed less favorably than other, less expressive winners. Observers also reported that they would be less likely to befriend these effusive winners than they would be to befriend the other winners, who were viewed as showing more appropriate humility.[32]

The situational constraints on positive emotion are also more pronounced following potential trauma. In one of our 9/11 studies, we asked New York college students to view either a sad film or an amusing film and then, afterward, to talk about what their lives had been like in the months after the attack. We filmed the students and later measured genuine smiles of happiness, coded from the muscles surrounding the eyes. Although, as in our previous research, genuine smiles overall predicted better future mental health, these benefits varied according to context. For students who watched the amusing film, smiling was unrelated to later mental health. This makes sense. Smiling is easy after watching something amusing, and thus should have no particular long-term benefit. But smiling is much more difficult when we are feeling down. Not surprisingly, students who watched the sad film felt a lot of negative emotion, but the more they smiled when talking about their lives afterward, the quicker that emotion dissipated. And, critically, smiling after the sad film also predicted better mental health two years later.[33]

But again, we come to the same refrain: not all aversive situations are the same, and no behavior, even smiling, is always adaptive. In another study, we examined genuine smiles of happiness in late adolescent girls as they described the most distressing experiences they had ever had. The girls who showed genuine smiles overall had better social adjustment two years later. But these effects varied depending on a key feature of the study: approximately half of the girls had documented histories of childhood sexual abuse, only they didn't know that we knew this. Thus, when we asked them to talk about their most distressing experience, they didn't have to disclose that they had been abused. And in fact, not all the sexually abused girls described their past abuse experience. But, crucially, if they did describe an abuse experience, expressing positive emotions in that context predicted worse, not better, social adjustment. Why? It's one thing for positive emotions to not always be useful, but why harmful?

The most likely explanation in this case had to do with the fact that sexual abuse is stigmatized. The disclosure of abuse tends to make people highly uncomfortable, and has even been known to evoke blame toward the survivor. Expressing positive emotion in such a loaded context would likely only make things worse or more confusing to listeners, or perhaps could even anger them. Although we can't know what their intentions might have been, the girls who smiled while disclosing past abuse probably had some difficulties detecting social cues about appropriate emotional expression, which no doubt contributed to their declining social adjustment.[34] This is an important point, and we'll come back to it a bit later.

Not Enough of a Bad Thing

What about the opposite: a behavior or trait nearly universally viewed as bad or unhealthy that is sometimes useful? Threat perception is a good example. We've already seen that trauma severity predicts reduced resilience, but only weakly. This showed us that there had to be more to it. Here, then, is another part of that story. The severity of a potential trauma depends not only on what happens to someone objectively, but also on how a person subjectively perceives the threat. The *subjective perception of threat* is, after all, a fundamental component of traumatic stress. It's also one of the primary reasons for saying an event is *potentially* traumatic rather than just plain traumatic.

Research bears this out. A large-scale study of traumatic injury patients found, for example, that one of the best predictors of later PTSD was the extent to which patients perceived their injuries to be life threatening. Similarly, in our own research, we found that people hospitalized for a possible heart attack who felt highly threatened when they first visited the emergency department were more likely to show enduring PTSD symptoms than patients who did not feel this level of threat. Patients who felt the lowest levels of threat perception were more likely to show a resilience trajectory. Importantly, these results were similar regardless of whether the patients were actually diagnosed with a heart attack. In other words, the perception of threat was at least as important as the actual objective level of threat.[35]

We saw this same basic result in our 9/11 research. In those studies, both the actual events people experienced—their objective exposure—and their subjective perceptions of personal risk predicted later PTSD symptoms. Critically, when we examined both simultaneously, we found that people who ultimately showed a resilience trajectory perceived themselves to be in relatively less danger at the time of the attacks regardless of their actual objective exposure.[36]

But, even these findings, or at least their apparent consistency, can be misleading. The personal risks evoked by potential trauma are multifaceted. They come and go and peak at different points before, during, and after the event itself. Given this kind of variability, as you can probably guess by now, the overall effects of risk perception, such as trauma severity, turn out to be relatively small, and to vary depending on context and timing. And, in many situations, threat perception is important, if not essential.

We get some clues as to why when we look more closely at how these perceptions are formed. The objective assessment of risk is relatively straightforward. Risk perception experts have honed the process down to four basic steps. They begin by first determining that threat is actually present; then, in sequence, they characterize its features, the level of exposure, and the overall level of risk. Nonexperts, which is the rest of us, tend to weigh risk more heavily in terms of our subjective emotional reactions—what experts call *risk as feelings*—and to rely on rapid, and largely unconscious, automatic processes geared toward immediate survival. One such process, harkening back to the type of mental shortcuts we discussed in Chapter 2, is to react quickly based on whatever partial information we have. We compare these limited perceptions against our memory of related experiences. If there is a match—and our previous experiences tell us we are in danger—we react with alarm. But if our associations in a given situation are not negative, or maybe even positive, we are likely to underestimate the possible risks involved and may fail to act with sufficient caution.[37] In other words, accurate threat perception is necessary for healthy adaptation.

The perils of threat underestimation are driven home poignantly in the context of sexual victimization. Although experts in this area are always concerned about blaming the victim, they nonetheless champion the fundamental importance of teaching girls and women to recognize and respond to risk. "One of the primary means a woman has at her disposal to reduce her risk for sexual assault," the experts advise, "is to learn to identify, and respond effectively to, risky situations that may increase her vulnerability to assault. Indeed, the earlier a woman is able to detect risk the more options available for her to escape a risky situation or, if necessary, mount an effective defense."[38]

A particularly tricky situation in this regard is when sexual assault happens with someone familiar to the victim, as, for example, in date rape. Sexual feelings with a known partner or acquaintance can often be pleasurable, and they can activate strong positive associations that lead an unsuspecting victim to ignore the danger cues. This can be an especially confusing scenario for women who've previously been sexually victimized. Researchers have studied the problem by asking women to listen to an audiotape of a simulated sexual encounter between a heterosexual couple as it rapidly evolves from affection to verbal coercion and then to threats of violence and ultimately rape. Their task in this case is to press a button when it appears that the date should be halted because the man depicted in the tape has "gone too far." Women who had repeatedly experienced sexual victimization had more difficulty decoding the cues and tended to halt the encounter later than other women in the study. They were also more likely to delay halting the date until the threat was painfully obvious (for example, there were verbal threats and use of force by the male protagonist, along with adamant refusals by the female, such as "Don't you dare touch me!" and "Get off me!"). Yet, somewhat ironically, even among women with previous sexual victimization, those with more PTSD arousal symptoms, which include hypervigilance to threat, but not other types of PTSD symptoms were quicker to perceive the danger cues and faster to signal the termination of the date compared to those who had fewer arousal symptoms.[39]

The real-world consequences of threat underestimation in sexual encounters are sobering. In another simulation study, regardless of whether the women in the study had previously experienced sexual victimization, both delayed threat detection and a delayed behavioral response to the threat predicted a greater likelihood of actual sexual victimization in the future, after the study had concluded.[40]

When we broaden our lens to other types of potential trauma, we find that the consequences of risk perception can vary depending on the context.[41] Following an urban terrorist attack, for example, people who thought a second terrorist attack might be imminent were more likely to engage in useful proactive behaviors, such as canceling plans, restricting destinations, or seeking contact and support from significant others, than those who perceived lower levels of threat. However, these responses varied depending on where the respondents lived in relation to the attack, their ages, and their genders.[42] Another study looked at survivors of floods. It found that people's fears about floods in general, as well as their assessments of how likely a future flood was in their region, could motivate them to prepare in appropriate ways for possible flooding. These factors, however, varied according to the survivors' emotional reactions to the previous flood as well as the severity of that flood.

In high-risk circumstances, reacting quickly to a threat can be essential for survival. This is true, for example, in dangerous professions, such as law enforcement. One study showed that threat perception among police trainees predicted how well they managed later in their careers as police officers. In this case, trainees who had a strong stress hormone release while viewing a distressing training film—indicating they were responsive to the threat—were more likely to show a resilience trajectory over the next four years. Trainees who had a more blunted response to the film—and thus were not responding to the threat—were more likely to show a trajectory of chronically increasing distress.[43]

Attention to threat can be especially important when high-risk events occur in contexts that are normally not associated with danger. One example is when civilians suddenly find themselves confronted with the terrifying threat of war. Researchers in Israel provided a compelling demonstration of this point by measuring attention to threat during a period of rocket attacks among residents of two different geographical regions: one that received heavy aerial attack and one that was under threat but not directly attacked. Predictably, attending to the level of the threat was not critical for residents of the region that was not actually attacked. In the heavily attacked area, however, paying attention to the threat was a matter of life or death. Among residents of this area, higher threat awareness showed a clear relationship to better mental health—specifically, less PTSD and depression one year later.[44] Again, timing also came into play. When the researchers repeated the measurements a year after the attacks had ceased, threat perception was inconsequential in both geographic regions.

Too much focus on threat at the wrong time can also be harmful. This can happen, for example, in life-threatening situations where staying focused on a threat has little or no clear function. A perfect example of this scenario comes from the heart attack study I mentioned a bit earlier. Threat perception was measured in this study while patients were in the emergency room. By that point, they had already responded to the threat signal from their bodies, which was how they got to the hospital in the first place. Once there, there was nothing more to do but remain as calm as possible and allow themselves to be cared for. A preoccupied focus on the threat at that point, when it was no longer useful, reduced the likelihood of resilience.[45]

The Right Behavior in the Right Situation at the Right Time

Most people manage to endure traumatic stress without serious or prolonged psychological harm. Most people are resilient. Yet, paradoxically, as we've seen, the traits and behaviors that correlate with resilience show pretty modest effects, and this is largely because no one trait or behavior is always useful. Every behavior, and every trait, comes with both benefits and costs. What works for one situation, one particular moment in time, may not work as well in another situation or at another moment in time. Putting it all together, we come to the unsurprising conclusion that since most people are resilient, most people must somehow work this out. Most people must be flexible enough to determine what the right behavior is in a given situation and at a given time, and then be able to engage in that behavior to adapt and move forward. If you have followed the story so far, this kind of flexibility should almost seem obvious. But, as we'll see shortly, there is a lot more to flexibility than meets the eye.

PART III

Getting Ourselves into the Game

CHAPTER 5

A Mindset for Flexibility

Flexibility is usually defined as having something to do with adapting, with being easily modified, bending but not breaking. The term is often used interchangeably with synonyms such as plasticity, pliability, adjustability, suppleness, give, and sometimes even resilience. But, just to be clear, flexibility and resilience are conceptually distinct. I've used the word "resilience" throughout this book to describe a pattern of continued good mental health after potential trauma, or, more precisely, *a stable trajectory of healthy functioning across time*. Flexibility is not resilience. Flexibility is the process we use to adapt ourselves to traumatic stress so that we can find our way to resilience.

At the core of this process is a series of steps I call *the flexibility sequence*. These are the nuts and bolts of flexibility. There is a lot that goes into the sequence, and in due course we will explore each step in some detail. But before we do that, we need to understand how it is that, in the face of adversity, we can motivate ourselves to carry out that process in the first place.

Flexibility does not simply happen. It is not a passive process. Although we often represent the idea of flexibility with images of some sort of pliable material, such as rubber or bamboo, that passively bends with pressure, humans do not simply bend. We bend ourselves. That process takes at least some effort and engagement with the task at hand.

The same is true of any skilled behavior. No matter how accomplished we might be, we still need to be motivated to put our skills to use. Top athletes and musicians, for example, may have all the right abilities but still not perform well if they don't have the right mindset, the right attitude and motivation to use their abilities. And like athletes and musicians, we cannot fully take advantage of our flexibility skills unless we first get our mind into the game. We need to have what I call a *flexibility mindset*.

A flexibility mindset is especially critical in the aftermath of a potentially traumatic event. These events are like shocks to the system. They have an immediacy, a sense of urgency and danger that sends the body's stress response into high gear. We saw this kind of intense, traumatic stress response in vivid detail as Will, Eva, and Reina wound their way through the labyrinth-like dangers they faced during the 9/11 attacks. The stress they experienced helped them to focus. It helped them find the energy to endure demanding physical challenges and, when necessary, to flee as fast as they could. But it also overwhelmed them at times. And unfortunately, in some cases, traumatic stress continues to overwhelm long after the event that instigated it has receded. When that happens, traumatic stress evolves, as it did for Will, into the more enduring and disabling set of difficulties typically described as PTSD.

Most of the time we are able to manage traumatic stress without serious or lasting harm. Even so, some of the more disturbing thoughts and images from the event will often linger for days or even weeks afterward. Usually, we want nothing more than to push these thoughts and images away. But, in order to do that, we need to pay attention. We need to take stock of what is happening to us and how we are reacting to it, at least long enough to understand what we can do about it. A flexibility mindset helps that process along.

The flexibility mindset is essentially a conviction that we will be able to adapt ourselves to the challenge at hand, that we will do whatever is needed to move forward. At the core of the mindset are three interrelated beliefs: *optimism* about the future, *confidence* in our ability to cope, and a willingness to think about a threat as a *challenge*. Each of these beliefs has been found, independently, to correlate with resilient outcomes. You've now heard repeatedly that the traits and behaviors associated with resilience correlate only modestly and are not effective in every situation. Thus, we know that optimism, confidence in coping, and a challenge orientation by themselves can't make us resilient. Nonetheless, the fact that they are correlated with resilience, even if modestly, tells us that at some point they must do something useful. Now we can begin to see what that something useful is.

Although individually each of these beliefs describes a generally healthy attitude, when they come together something else happens, something larger. These beliefs interact and complement each other in a way that multiplies their individual impact. And collectively they produce a robust conviction, a mindset, that says, in effect, "I will not fail. I will find a way to deal with this challenge." There may be other means to generate the motivation we need to get ourselves into the game and respond flexibly. But none that I know of is as straightforward, or as powerful, as the collective impact of these three beliefs.

The concept of a flexibility mindset owes a clear debt to several related concepts—for example, a growth mindset, along with its opposite, a fixed mindset, developed by psychologist Carol Dweck. Originally conceived as a way to help foster student learning, the growth-versus-fixed mindset concept goes something like this: People who struggle to learn new ideas or skills often fail because they believe that the talent they need for those ideas or skills is innate. You either have it or you don't. This is called a fixed mindset, and it is often reinforced by common educational practices, such as intelligence testing. When students who've developed a fixed mindset do poorly, it only seems to confirm their mindset. Often, they simply give up and stop trying. They tell themselves, "Why bother? If people are either talented or not, and I have failed, then I must not have much talent." By contrast, students who believe, or can be convinced, that talent is malleable, that they can improve—say, through hard work, perseverance, or useful guidance from others—develop a growth mindset. These students tend to do better over time. They keep trying and eventually master the needed skills.

A flexibility mindset is not the same as a growth mindset, but there are obvious similarities. Like the growth mindset, a flexibility mindset involves the conviction that it is possible to master a challenge. But by the same token, as Dweck is quick to point out, "people often confuse a growth mindset with being flexible or open-minded or with having a positive outlook," qualities that clearly resonate with the flexibility mindset.[1] Her main point of contention, though, is not so much with the idea that these qualities are incompatible with growth, but with the assumption that such qualities are innate traits, something we either have or don't have. Here, again, we find resonance with the flexibility mindset. Although the beliefs that make up a flexibility mindset do appear to be somewhat trait-like, they are in fact malleable, and, as we will find in later chapters, they can be cultivated and enhanced.

The idea of a flexibility mindset also harkens back to an earlier and now nearly forgotten concept known as *stress hardiness*.[2] Originally proposed in the late 1970s by Suzanne Kobasa (now Ouellette-Kobasa) and her mentor Salvador Maddi, stress hardiness revolves around three beliefs: a sense of commitment to the tasks of one's life, a feeling of control, and a willingness to embrace stressors as challenges. The first two beliefs are only loosely similar to optimism and confidence in coping, while the third, challenge orientation, maps closely to the challenge orientation of the flexibility mindset.

When the hardiness concept first appeared, it stimulated a great deal of new thinking about how mindset and coping interacted. But gradually, as researchers questioned whether hardiness actually buffered against stress, it fell out of favor. The demotion was premature. Hardiness had been forgotten not because it wasn't useful, but because, like a growth mindset, it was easily misconstrued as a type, in this case a hardiness type.[3] That was a wrong turn, and unfortunately it led to a great deal of misunderstanding and misuse of the concept.

Ouellette-Kobasa and Maddi were cleverer than that. They did not see hardiness as a type. Nor did they view its components as buffering stress or producing resilience. Rather, they wisely saw hardiness as an intermediate step, a collection of beliefs that "provides the courage and motivation to do the hard work of turning stressful circumstances from potential disasters into growth opportunities." This set of beliefs, they said, creates a "pathway" that can eventually lead to resilience.[4]

The flexibility mindset builds on this same seminal idea.[5] Just as hardiness by itself does not buffer against stress, the flexibility mindset by itself doesn't make us resilient. But it does pave the way for resilience by motivating us and engaging us with the stressor. It enables us to do "the hard work" of flexibly adapting ourselves to the challenges we face.

Early Clues

Although we haven't discussed the details of the flexibility mindset until now, we saw hints of it earlier when Jed was about to go into surgery. In that moment, Jed seemed unusually calm, and he briefly but clearly expressed optimism and confidence about his recovery, both components of a flexibility mindset.

Signs of a flexibility mindset were also evident in Reina's 9/11 account, not in her narrative about the day of the attack—there was simply too much going on that day, and at that point she was preoccupied with survival—but later, when we asked her and other survivors about their experiences in the weeks following the attacks.

Once she was home safely, Reina was finally reunited with her husband and children. Initially, she told us, she was nearly overwhelmed by traumatic stress. But as she shared her experiences with an ever-changing mix of concerned family and friends, their support buffeted her. Fairly early on, she felt confident that she would be able to cope with her intrusive memories. Despite the fact that she frequently thought and dreamt about the attacks, she was certain she would find a way to manage them. "I'm not sure why," she told us. "But I had the sense that I could handle this."

Reina also showed signs of a challenge orientation. Although she was comfortable with other people, she nonetheless anticipated that there were likely to be at least a few difficult social situations ahead, and she planned how she might best address those challenges. She made sure, for example, to get herself out of the house and around other people so that she could test the waters. As life began to return to normal, she was able to more fully engage with other people without much difficulty.

She also thought about how she might find a way to travel when she had to. Like other survivors, after the attacks Reina was uneasy traveling by plane. It was such a poignant reminder. But she traveled by plane anyway. As she put it, "I wasn't thrilled, but I did it. I got through it." One of the solutions Reina hit upon—again, using her social aplomb—was to talk with her fellow passengers. "I am a social person, but I don't usually talk much on planes. I like my privacy. But after 9/11, it was, well, you know I was anxious about travel and so I talked to people, anyone, anyone within earshot. It helped. I'm not sure why, but since it seemed to make it easier, I kept doing it."

During the course of our interview with Reina, we also discovered that she was deliberately trying to maintain an optimistic outlook. Although we didn't ask directly about optimism, we did routinely ask survivors whether they could imagine or look forward to a positive future.

"Do I look forward to the future? Yeah, I usually do. I kept telling myself, 'It will be okay, this is going to pass, just remember the good in your life,' and I kind of made myself think about what I would be doing in the future, even if, you know, because everything was in flux after the attack, I wasn't exactly sure what that would be. . . . But now I am busy, and I am excited about new projects. Everything is basically okay. I'm happy. I am looking forward to whatever comes next."

In the pages ahead, we will explore each of these beliefs—optimism, confidence in coping, and a challenge orientation—and show how they interact and reinforce each other to create a flexibility mindset. Optimism is probably the best known of the three. We'll begin there.

Optimism

In the psychological literature, optimism is defined as a general belief that the future will turn out well, even when there is no particular evidence that this is likely to be the case. In other words, optimism is a bias, an interpretation of possible futures that is tilted toward the positive. Not surprisingly, some people are reliably more optimistic than others.[6] But almost everyone is capable of being optimistic at least some of the time.

The idea that optimism promotes resilience has circulated for some time in popular books and in the media.[7] It's also supported by quite a bit of research evidence. People who score well on measures of optimism on average do cope well with aversive or potentially traumatic life events. My own research has shown that optimistic people are more likely than non-optimists to evidence the resilience trajectory following a potentially traumatic event. In one study, we showed that optimism, measured years before a potentially traumatic event, predicted a resilience trajectory once that event occurred.[8]

These findings harken back again to the resilience paradox.[9] Nobody is optimistic all the time or in every situation. Relentless optimism would actually be unrealistic, if not downright delusional. And, like virtually all of the predictors of resilient outcomes, sometimes optimism is not effective. Sometimes it can even lead to a worse outcome.[10] Yet optimism is still beneficial when it comes to helping us cope with potential trauma—not because a person is optimistic all the time, or because optimism makes a person resilient, but because optimism motivates us to work for that expected positive future as part of the flexibility mindset. Whether or not a resilient outcome actually comes to pass, of course, depends, as we will see shortly, on more than optimism.

•

MAREN WAS A generally optimistic person. She grew up in Düsseldorf, Germany, and, although her childhood was fairly typical of middle-class Germans, it was clear early on that she was intelligent and talented, especially when it came to language. After completing high school, like many of her friends she prepared to go abroad for a "gap year" before beginning university. Her English was already quite advanced, and when an opportunity presented itself to spend the year in London, she leapt at the chance. Near the end of her first year she decided to apply for study at the prestigious University of Cambridge. To her delight, she was accepted. She had just turned twenty-one, and her future couldn't have been rosier.

One weekend, during her second year at Cambridge, a fellow student invited Maren to join him for a trip to the countryside. He kept a horse in Wiltshire, a region famous for its ancient archeological sites. They could stay in a bed and breakfast, he suggested, explore the countryside, and do some riding. Maren remembers thinking it all sounded so very romantic.

Wiltshire has a relatively more temperate climate than other parts of England, and the first day of their visit was perfect for riding. They decided to go directly to the stables, but when they arrived they discovered that only one horse was available.

Undaunted, the couple decided they could still make a day of it if they took turns with the one horse. Maren's companion went first, and then, when it was Maren's turn, her companion rode along on a bicycle.

Maren had always loved horses. As a child, she had taken riding lessons, and she had even learned some acrobatic vaulting techniques. Although she didn't consider herself an experienced rider, she thought she could handle a horse reasonably well.

Riding a new horse for the first time is always a bit challenging. And on top of it, this particular horse had also been suffering from a painful bone disease and hadn't been exercised for some time. Maren knew none of this. Her only thoughts were that the day was looking gorgeous, she was with a potential new boyfriend, and she was going to be riding again.

They set off with smiles on their faces.

At first, they ambled at a slow gait, Maren on the horse, her friend on the bicycle, talking and enjoying the beautiful weather. Eventually they came to an open field and Maren signaled the horse to trot. The reason for what happened next, whether it was the horse's pain, or his displeasure about having a new rider, was never clear. The horse bolted and bucked, and threw Maren off.

It happened so quickly. One moment she felt herself sliding; the next she found herself lying flat on her back in the grass. When she tried to get up, she found she couldn't move.

•

THE SPINAL CORD is the primary conduit of the central nervous system, a superhighway that carries sensory and motor information to and from the brain. Its network of nerve fibers links up just about every part of our bodies, and it plays a huge role in much of what we normally do without our even noticing: breathing, moving, digesting, experiencing physical sensation, responding sexually. The information transmitted along the spine is so crucial that it's the only part of the nervous system other than the brain that gets its own protective bone casing.

Injuries to the spinal cord are always serious. The best one can hope for is that the spinal tissue is only bruised. Bruising causes minor nerve damage and a temporary loss of feeling in a circumscribed part of the body, such as a hand or a foot. Unfortunately, more intense, traumatic impacts can shatter vertebrae and puncture or even sever the cord. When this happens, the damage is often permanent and results in varying degrees of paralysis. *Paraplegia* refers to the loss of sensory or motor functioning in the lower extremities. *Tetraplegia*, or *quadriplegia*, is a paralysis of all the limbs and torso. Serious spinal cord injuries are not always so easily categorized, however, and survivors often describe their condition in more informative terms regarding the location of their injury, the specific vertebrae. The higher up along the spinal column, the greater the loss of bodily functioning.

•

MAREN LAY FROZEN in the field where only minutes ago she had been carefree and enjoying the blossoming day. What must have been going through her mind? As she remembers it, she was not at all sure what had happened.

"I was not aware. I didn't really understand. All I knew was I was holding on and then I was sliding, and the next thing I knew I was on my back and I can't get up, and I don't know why."

Fortunately, she was not alone. Even more fortunate, there was a hospital nearby that specialized in the treatment of spinal cord injury. Maren was transported there by helicopter.

She tried to remain calm, but when she arrived at the hospital, fear began to overtake her.

"What was scary was it seemed like I was being moved around forever, through all these corridors in this hospital, and x-rayed left and right. I was in a lot of pain. All this time I kept thinking: give me some medications. I want to be out of this."

Maren's family was in Germany. When her mother learned of the injury, she flew to England and arrived the next day. Maren was still finding it difficult to fully grasp the severity of her situation.

"I had not realized what had happened to me. It did not occur to me that I had a spinal cord injury. The weird thing is that I was still concerned with really silly things. Like, this guy I had met was a new romantic interest and I was still thinking about that. What would he think? It was ridiculous. Here I had this really intense injury, yet I had no idea what it really meant. I lacked any sense of proportion of what had happened to me."

That all began to change when Maren and her mother finally had a chance to talk.

The German word for paraplegia due to spinal cord injury is *Querschnittslähmung*. She knew the word in German and English. But the English phrase *spinal cord lesion* did not yet carry the same serious connotations for her. When she spoke with her mother in German, and heard *Querschnittslähmung*, it finally sank in.

Maren's memory of that moment is indelible.

"I thought, 'Oh my God.'"

A spinal cord injury is life changing. If it wasn't yet clear to Maren exactly how her world was going to change, she had to be thinking that whatever happened, it was going to be bad—impossibly bad. Probably the worst thing she'd ever experienced.

The injury fractured Maren's thoracic vertebrae in four areas. This was extremely worrisome. The thoracic region is relatively high up in the spinal column. Fortunately, Maren's injury had not severed her spinal cord. That, at least, was good news. A severed spine is all but impossible to repair. Nonetheless, her spinal cord seemed to be seriously damaged, and the prognosis was not good.

One of the common medical procedures for cases like Maren's is to surgically insert metal rods to help support the weakened spinal structure. This would allow the spine to endure greater stress and make possible at least some mobility. The hospital surgeon who normally would have done this was away for the Easter holiday. In his stead, an older, more conservative doctor treated Maren. He decided against the surgery. And without the metal supports, it would be necessary for Maren to lie as still as possible day and night for nine long weeks. The only movement she would experience would be when the nurses came to turn her body to prevent skin pressure sores.

Lying immobile, helpless in her hospital bed, there wasn't much Maren could do except think. How could she not help but conjure images of a depressing future? What if she never walked again? She couldn't imagine returning to her former life at Cambridge in a wheelchair. Even the thought of doing so was "extremely scary and depressing."

Most of us have suffered the weight of deep sadness at some point in our lives. A major depressive episode is far worse. Major depression is insidious. It doesn't appear suddenly, like the flu, or a muscle cramp. It festers. The symptoms feed off each other. They gather steam, and gradually they spiral into a deeper and deeper malaise.

A full-blown depression has two hallmark symptoms. One is a sad or depressed mood that persists throughout most of the day for a continual period of time. The second is a loss of interest in the things that one would normally find engaging or pleasurable. When depression spins out of control, these two symptoms are accompanied by other problems: difficulty thinking or concentrating, fatigue, poor sleep or excessive need to sleep, feelings of worthlessness, and noticeable changes in appetite. Depression also tends to co-occur with symptoms of anxiety—in particular, excessive worry and apprehension.

Even if Maren could somehow manage to keep depressing, anxious thoughts at bay, there was still the injury itself. By nearly any standard, Maren's fall and its aftermath would have been traumatic. Sudden, life threatening, and painful, it was the perfect recipe for PTSD.[11]

When the spinal cord is injured, a period of spinal shock ensues, usually lasting several weeks, in which the nerve fibers are either completely or partially unresponsive. This is a risky period and in extreme cases can result in cardiac arrest or other dangerous failures of the autonomic nervous system. There may be headaches, too, or odd sensations and excessive sweating.

During these initial days, Maren did her best to banish whatever frantic, dreadful thoughts were hovering around her hospital bed. She was heavily sedated with morphine to reduce the pain. That certainly helped. But, although Maren was generally an optimistic person, she couldn't assume everything was simply going to be fine on its own. A spinal cord injury is a very serious matter, and at this point she was acutely aware of that fact. She did everything she could to keep her spirits up. Using whatever energy she could muster, she focused her thoughts, deliberately and unceasingly, on one goal: getting better. She was adamant about this. She was not going to give in.

"I just wasn't buying into the story. I could not accept that I was not going to walk again."

Maren discovered that music was a great help. She found it transported her, and that she could use it to conjure positive images of health.[12]

"I imagined myself healed and able to walk. I imagined walking along a beach."

Maren's mother and brothers—who had also flown to England—shared her belief in the value of optimism. They reinforced it any way they could. This was an enormous boost for Maren. They brought her music. They rubbed her legs. Whatever might work, they were willing to try it.

The story was a bit different with Maren's father. He was an active man, and he meant well, and no sooner than he arrived from Germany, he threw himself into Maren's situation. But for him, helping was not about good vibes, it was about details and facts. He busied himself gathering as much information as he could on the ins and outs of spinal cord injury and about Maren's care.

If there was anything to be gained from knowing more, at this early juncture Maren was not interested. "I tried not to expose myself to too much information," she recalls. "That was not part of my plan. I tried only to focus on positive thoughts about healing, not details about my injury."

In the first days after an injury, it is usually not yet clear how much functioning might be recovered. Only when the initial spinal shock begins to subside does it become possible to more clearly determine the severity of the injury and how well or how poorly the patient might cope with it.

For Maren, that turning point came ten days after the injury. The spinal shock appeared to be lifting.

And then it happened.

"I moved my toes. . . . Sensation was slowly coming back."

She was thrilled.

Her family and friends were excited for her as well.

She had only moved her toes a tiny bit, a few millimeters. But those few millimeters seemed huge.

"When I moved my toes, it was a big deal. It could have meant nothing, but I had something to build on. I became completely convinced I would walk again."

Not everyone shared in the elation, or in Maren's optimism. Her doctors had seen this before. They were extremely cautious, if not downright pessimistic. A little movement of a toe, they told Maren, was exciting but not really meaningful. They had looked closely at her data, and they still thought, unfortunately, that the prognosis was dire.

One reason for their pessimism was that they knew spinal shock does more than numb physical sensation. It can impact how patients experience the first days of their injury. The interruption of signaling to the brain may impair thought processes, flatten emotions, or make it harder for patients to grasp what has happened to them. In later stages of spinal shock, some physicians have noted, patients may appear to be surprisingly cooperative or even cheerful, and their mood and interactions with hospital staff are appropriate and normal. But don't take this stage too seriously, they warn, for the apparent normal emotional adjustment these patients show is probably deceptive. They will soon begin to experience a period of anger, and then, once they realize the full extent of their situation, undoubtedly, they will begin to show signs of distress and depression.[13]

Motivation

When Maren moved her toes, she felt "electrified." This was all the proof she needed. She had been working hard to maintain an optimistic stance. Now she felt her optimism soar.

But would it make any difference? Her prognosis was dire. Could her rosy view of the future really do much good? Could she use it to repel the looming sense of hopelessness and despair that was all around her and keep her sights on recovery?

One thing an optimistic, future-oriented bias can do exceptionally well is motivate. Adapting to any adverse situation is work, and staying focused on that work requires fuel. Believing in an optimistic future provides just the right motivational thrust to give us that fuel. When research participants were asked to imagine positive future events in an fMRI scanner, they showed greater activation in the amygdala, an area associated with evaluation of the emotional significance of an event, and in the rostral anterior cingulate cortex, an area associated with, among other things, emotional decision-making and anticipation of future rewards. When we imagine positive future events, these two areas of the brain share strong reciprocal neural connections. They appear to work in concert to help us anticipate when the future will bring us something good, thus motivating us to engage with that future. People who score high on measures of optimism show these same rewarding-future brain activation patterns to an even stronger degree.[14]

Optimism makes us willing to do the work needed to reach that positive future. Just about anything we do requires energy and effort. When we physically exert ourselves, we burn calories, and as anyone who uses a step tracker or Fitbit-type device knows, the more we move or the harder we work out, the more calories we burn. The same is true, generally, for brain activity. Our brains are constantly working, even when we are at rest, and brain activity requires a surprisingly large portion of our available metabolic resources. How we think about the world influences just about everything we do, and it is intimately related to how much effort we might expend and how much energy we need. Thinking hard and long about emotionally demanding topics requires even more resources, and the effect often extends to other bodily functions, such as the release of stress hormones and increases in heart rate. Although we haven't yet gotten into the details, thinking flexibly also involves energy and effort. When people feel optimistic, they are more likely to devote energy and effort to working on their problems; they assume that the future will be good and that it is worth the exertion.[15]

In the same way, an optimistic anticipation of a rewarding future has a self-fulfilling quality to it. Optimists are proactive about taking care of themselves. And, not surprisingly, they tend to be healthier than other people and to live longer.[16] Because optimists believe they will be successful, they tend to be more persistent in the endeavors they take on. At least in part for this reason, they are actually more successful. The same holds true in the social world. Optimists tend to have better and closer relationships than non-optimists, again probably for the same self-fulfilling reasons.[17]

.

MAREN WAS THRILLED when she moved her toes. But she had a tough road ahead. She still had to deal with the ongoing physical pain. The first week after the spinal shock subsided was particularly trying. When the spine is injured, the link between the brain and the motor neurons that govern muscle action is broken. In a sense, the motor neurons begin to function independently. Because they are no longer directly linked to the brain, they often fire spontaneously, causing waves of intense muscle spasm.[18] The pain was excruciating. To weaken the spasms, Maren had to force herself as best she could to relax her body. At times it was rough going, but her family was with her, and she endured it as best she could. Eventually, as the motor pathways healed, the spasms gradually subsided. All the while, Maren never allowed her optimism to lag.

"I had set myself this goal: I was going to walk again. That goal was what my life revolved around for the next two years."

Propelled by her optimism, she thought carefully about how she would achieve her goal. Then, she dug in for the long haul.

Not surprisingly, the tenacity of her belief that she would walk again sometimes meant that she had to butt heads with a medical establishment that assumed she was either in denial or just plain foolish.

Maren remembers one particular stressful memory of this sort. Around six weeks after the injury, it was decided that she should return to Germany so she could be treated closer to her family. This was not a simple endeavor, as it would require a plane ride. To avoid further injury, Maren had to be completely immobilized during the flight. She prepared herself and did her best to keep her spirits up.

"I would sort of flirt and chat with the emergency people who were escorting me on the plane. We were having this fun conversation. But then they looked at my records, and they began to treat me differently afterward. They became quite serious."

She asked them if she might see her records. She had not until that point actually read her medical charts. It was an especially difficult moment.

"The records were very negative, basically predicting that I would be wheelchair bound. The language they used was . . . well . . . shocking. I was always trying to be very positive, but the language in the records was so negative."

The disparity only grew worse. Maren had always found the British doctors to be overly cautious. But when she was transferred to a German hospital, she discovered that the German doctors were even more conservative.

"The German doctors were very negative about my chances of ever walking again."

Yet, Maren persevered in the optimistic belief that she would regain at least some aspects of a normal life, and she stayed focused on that belief.

The first hospital in Germany had an outstanding reputation as a research facility, but Maren never felt comfortable there. She decided she should move to a hospital that might be more amenable to her positive approach and lobbied to be relocated.

Eventually, she found a hospital that seemed a better fit and was able to arrange to be transferred there.

Costs?

Could there be a downside to Maren's steadfast optimism? As we've seen, like any resilience-promoting factor, optimism isn't always helpful and, in some situations, it may even be harmful. For example, optimism can lead to overly positive expectations that may, in the end, only result in crushing disappointment. Optimism can also lead to unrealistic hope for a desired outcome that may be highly unlikely, as is sometimes the case in cancer treatments. Physicians report that many patients begin treatment with unrealistically high expectations. One study, for example, found that the majority of treatment-seeking cancer patients believed that their personal chances of benefiting from treatment were greater, and their risk lower, than they were for the average person.[19] Nonetheless, even in dire circumstances, if we separate the likelihood of an unwanted outcome from our expectations of how well we actually cope with its aftermath, optimism can still be salubrious. In fact, research has shown that even when facing the formidable threat of cancer treatment, optimism still helps people manage the stress of that treatment.[20]

•

ONCE SHE SETTLED into the new, more sympathetic hospital, Maren immediately turned her attention to strengthening her body.

"I really threw myself into the medical regime. I did everything I could. I took advantage of everything the hospital had to offer me. I went above and beyond. I went to the gym outside of hours, and did weights by myself."

Although she still used a wheelchair, she had begun to practice a kind of proto-walking using a combination of crutches and knee braces. Her condition improved markedly and, along with it, her ability to sustain her optimistic stance. She never stopped focusing on a positive future, never stopped believing she would recover the ability to walk and that everything would eventually work out for her. And fueled by her burgeoning optimism, she had an almost limitless capacity to try new approaches. She was open to literally any and all options that might promote recovery. Of course, sometimes this openness led her down blind alleys.

She laughs when she remembers.

"After you have an injury like this, everyone wants to heal you."

But there was also hope in new methods. While she was still in England, Maren's mother had brought her a book by American psychiatrist Gerald Jampolsky that told numerous inspirational stories of people who were able to overcome dire illness and injury by changing their beliefs.[21] Maren felt so hopeful when she read it that she wrote Jampolsky in the hopes of meeting with him. Not long after, back in Germany, Maren's family doctor had told her about a Hawaiian traditional healer, a *kahuna*, who used a form of massage called *lomilomi* to help people overcome serious physical impairment. The kahuna happened to be lecturing in Germany at the time, and the family doctor arranged for Maren to meet with him. Maren found him to be wonderfully "charismatic" and thought his approach would be helpful. During a casual conversation, the kahuna's apprentice suggested that Maren visit the Hawaiian island of Maui where he worked. Maren remembers thinking that it sounded like a genuine healing place.

Maui is a long way from Germany for a person with limited mobility. The trip would be expensive and difficult. It would require lots of advance planning. And it was still only a hopeful possibility. Nothing was guaranteed.

Most people would have probably dropped the idea right then and there. But Maren found the option deeply appealing and stayed in contact with the kahuna's team. As her legs grew stronger, she eventually did what she had to do to make the trip. Fortuitously, around this same time, Gerald Jampolsky had also written back to Maren. As it turned out, he and his wife and collaborator, Dr. Diane Cirincione, were also spending time in Hawaii, on one of the other islands, and they would be glad to meet with her.

Right from the start, Maren's experience of working with the kahuna and meeting with Jerry and Diane was exceedingly positive. So much so that, although she had originally planned to stay in Hawaii for six weeks, she ended up extending her trip to four months.

"I would have stayed longer if I could have," she laughs.

While in Hawaii, Maren exercised as much as possible. She swam in the ocean daily to build up her muscle strength. She also made many friends during this time and had what she remembers to be wonderfully meaningful discussions with Jerry, Diane, and other new friends.

Above all, Maren found a perfect match for her own relentlessly optimistic attitude.

"I loved it. People were so positive. I really love this about Americans. They have all these stories, almost fantasies, about people overcoming adversity. Americans love these kinds of stories. And they loved my story and encouraged me. It was a very positive time in my life."

Her progress was steady. And with each advance, her confidence was bolstered.

On the one-year anniversary of the accident, Maren traveled with a friend to the summit of the Haleakala crater on Maui to watch the sunrise. Later that afternoon, she and her friend went to the beach, and Maren tried for the first time to walk entirely on her own.

And she did it!

It was a hard-won fight, a very special moment, and a truly amazing victory.

But Maren was not done yet.

She kept working and strengthening her body and, two years after the injury, returned to the University of Cambridge to resume her studies. For Maren this was the ultimate triumph. She walked again on that campus, on her own two feet with no external aids. She was quietly proud of her accomplishment, but she deserved the cheers of a stadium crowd.

CHAPTER 6

Synergy

Years later, with the injury behind her, Maren came to appreciate why her doctors had been so cautious. Many people who suffer spinal cord lesions do regain some feeling, but often that's as far as it goes. For many spinal cord injury survivors, walking remains only a dream.

Maren eventually realized how unusual her physical recovery had been. She worked hard, that's undeniable. But there was also some luck in it. Optimism cannot mend a spinal cord that won't be mended. Maren's injury had to have been just within that narrow window of possibility for recovery. What if that window had not been there? What if her spine had not healed?

Maren has often contemplated this possibility. She wonders how well she would have coped if she had not been able to move her toes so soon after the injury, or if she never regained the ability to walk. She wonders if her optimism would have given way to despair.

This is where the other two beliefs that contribute to a flexibility mindset come into play. If Maren had relied solely on optimism, she may actually have succumbed. Optimism by itself is simply not enough. Focusing on a rosy future is without a doubt a powerful motivator, one that helps engage us to strive toward flexible solutions. But achieving that task, finding those flexible solutions, becomes much more difficult, if not impossible, if we rely solely on optimism, especially when the bad news just keeps coming.

I mentioned earlier that a flexibility mindset centers on the conviction that we will be able to adapt ourselves to the challenge at hand and do whatever is necessary to move forward. Optimism certainly contributes to that conviction. But something else happens when we add the other two parts of the mindset to the picture—confidence in coping and challenge orientation. These elements provide the extra thrust we need to confront difficult challenges, and as we'll see a bit later, they do more even than that.

Confidence and Challenge

Several years ago, I was participating in a symposium on resilience and serious adversity at a conference in Chicago.[1] There I met the late Paul Kennedy of Oxford University, at the time one of the world's leading experts on the psychology of spinal cord injury. After the panel, I shared a drink with Paul. He told me he was excited about the trajectory approach I had developed, and after a lengthy discussion, and a few more drinks, we decided we would test whether the same trajectories I had seen in my trauma research might also apply to data that Paul and his colleagues had collected on spinal cord injury. This was going to be a severe test. All the spinal cord patients in Paul's data had suffered the very outcome that Maren had so narrowly escaped. None of the patients in his study had moved their toes, or if they had, it didn't make any difference. They were all still paralyzed.

When we finally completed the study, the results were striking. Despite the severe nature of their injuries, we found, as we had in so many previous studies, that most of the spinal cord patients showed a clear resilience trajectory.[2] This was not a transient stage before the depressing reality set in. The resilient group had consistently low symptom levels even in the hospital, soon after their injury, and again each time they were assessed over the next several years. Even more striking, the resilient survivors' symptom levels were about the same as in the normal population. In other words, although they had been severely injured and paralyzed, the majority were no more depressed and no more anxious than the average person off the street. This was true even in the first weeks after the injury. But there was even more. The results of this study and others that followed showed that resilient survivors had all the ingredients of a flexibility mindset. They were optimistic, they saw themselves as efficacious copers, and they were fully focused on the challenges that lay before them.[3]

Confidence in coping motivates in a different way from optimism. It can give us that little extra push we need to be more adventurous. When we feel confident that we can handle ourselves, we will likely try a broader range of behaviors. We might even try behaviors we are not sure we are able to do, simply because we assume ourselves likely to succeed. And, like optimism, this kind of confidence becomes a self-fulfilling prophecy. People who view themselves as effective copers don't just think they cope better; on the whole they actually do cope better, both with current stressors and with whatever stressors they might encounter in the future. They also cope especially well in the aftermath of potentially traumatic events.[4] In a study we conducted on hospitalized survivors of traumatic injuries, for example, those who believed themselves to be efficacious copers at the time of hospitalization were more likely to show a resilience trajectory over the ensuing six months.[5]

A challenge orientation adds something a bit different to the mix. Probably the best way to get at the nature of this belief is to compare it with its opposite, a threat orientation. When people are confronted with serious adversity, it is only natural to feel threatened and, at least initially, to focus on how bad things might get.

As psychologists describe it, we make threat appraisals when "the perception of danger exceeds the perception of abilities or resources to cope with the stressor."[6] In other words, we expect that we are likely to be overwhelmed, or that we will be worse off because of the stressor than we were before. In essence, we are telling ourselves, "This is going to be bad, and it will probably get worse. I don't think I can handle it." The more we stay focused on the threat, the more likely we are to become distressed and anxious. Distressing, anxious emotions, in turn, often get in the way of our ability to take effective action. An enduring threat orientation fosters passive responding. We let the event happen to us rather than actively confronting it or trying to do something about it. And when we do that, we are less able to improve our situation.

When we shift our focus to the challenge, things begin to happen. For starters, we take a more active stance, and we begin to think about the stressor differently. We see it less as a threat to endure and more as a challenge to be met. In other words, when we embrace a challenge, we shift from simply telling ourselves how bad it is going to be to focusing on what we need to do to get past it.

A nice example of the way the challenge orientation promotes flexibility appeared in a recent news story about the iconoclastic composer John Zorn. Zorn had labored for months on a massive retrospective of his compositions. He supervised every aspect of the project, including lining up scores of musicians, recording them in various combinations for different pieces, and mixing the sound from the sessions to produce the final musical products. Then, just as the entire project was nearing completion, the financial backing fell through. It had been an enormously expensive project, and now there was no money to pay for any of it. After first absorbing this threat, "the initial shock," Zorn saw he had no choice but to shift gears. "I went into my let's-fix-it mode," he said. "I always have a Plan B. I try to find a way to solve the problem that's a creative way."[7]

In part, the adaptive changes brought about by a challenge orientation happen automatically in the way our bodies respond. A compelling series of laboratory studies demonstrated how this works. In one set of studies, people were asked how they thought they would react to a pending stressor situation, such as a mild electric shock. In another set, they were instructed to think about the stressor specifically as either a threat or a challenge. Regardless of whether they did so naturally or were instructed to do so, those who viewed the stressor as a challenge rather than a threat consistently exhibited bodily reactions that were more clearly geared toward action and adaptation.[8]

That adaptive response goes something like this. First, the sympathetic nervous system ramps up our cardiovascular response. There is greater ventricular contraction and enhanced cardiac output. Simply put, our hearts pump more blood. At the same time, the body releases the hormone epinephrine—more commonly known as adrenaline—into the bloodstream. Adrenaline promotes vasodilation in the large skeletal muscles and in the lungs, which in turn helps to keep blood pressure in check and prepares us to respond with greater energy and bodily resources. A longer-lasting and more powerful stress hormone, cortisol, may also be released, but this response is regulated, and we quickly adapt to it. Together, this suite of bodily reactions is comparable to those that occur during physical exercise when we are actively engaged and our bodies are performing well.

When we focus exclusively on the threat, by contrast, we again have the increased cardiovascular output, but without the accompanying vasodilation. Without this hormonal braking mechanism, enhanced cardiac output tends to result in excessively high blood pressure and a more enduring overall stress response.[9] And it does not trigger the physical preparedness we see with challenge appraisals. Indeed, the physiological responses to a threat orientation have been shown to be similar to the kind of passive stress response that happens when people immerse a hand or foot in ice-cold water.[10] In other words, there is passive endurance, and, as the pain worsens, our only recourse is to withdraw from it.

The orientation toward challenge becomes even more crucial when stressors persist over longer periods of time. For example, children who are bullied in school but interpret the situation as a challenge have been found to be more likely to seek help, and thus are more likely to overcome these experiences. Combat-deployed soldiers who show a generally healthy profile have been found to be more likely to view their experiences as challenges, and soldiers who are oriented this way are less depressed, have fewer physical complaints, and have less negative emotion and more positive emotion than other soldiers.[11]

A challenge orientation is especially adaptive for the kind of prolonged ordeal that spinal cord injury survivors have to endure. Paul Kennedy liked to tell a story about one of his spinal cord injury patients, a bricklayer who was paralyzed in his late twenties after a work-related injury. Rather than wallowing in self-pity, the bricklayer reinterpreted his misfortune as a challenge. Seeing it as an opportunity to refocus his life, he began taking courses at a local university. Along the way he discovered a deep love of statistics, and eventually he found his way to an exciting new career as a well-respected computational researcher. Although this outcome puts a happy ending to an otherwise tragic story, our bricklayer-turned-researcher took it further: he went as far as to say that his spinal cord injury was the best thing that ever happened to him. In telling this story, Paul always hastened to add, in his heavy Irish brogue, that "a little career counseling would have been easier."[12]

The links between the challenge orientation and psychological health are also readily apparent in Paul's research with large groups of spinal cord injury survivors. In one study, for example, survivors who had a challenge orientation were less depressed and less anxious than other survivors.[13] Similarly, in the trajectory study we jointly conducted, the spinal cord injury survivors who had a challenge orientation were more likely to be in the resilience trajectory than in other trajectories.[14] In that same study, resilient survivors scored highly on a related measure called "fighting spirit."[15] The questions used to rate this measure were tailored specifically to spinal cord injury survivors and showed an obvious affinity for a flexibility mindset—for example, they were asked if they agreed with statements such as "I try to make the best of my life despite the lesion," "I refuse to let the lesion rule my life," and "I always try to find tricks that might make my situation less difficult."

More Than the Sum of Its Parts

The three beliefs that contribute to the flexibility mindset are similar in many ways. Yet each one adds something unique to the mix. Optimism motivates us to work for a positive future. A challenge orientation gets us thinking about what it is that we need to do, and confidence in coping helps us do it. Although these are undeniable benefits, there are also potential costs, just as there are with virtually any other trait or behavior. We've already discussed the possible downside of excessive optimism. Confidence in coping and the challenge orientation also have potential shortcomings. For example, people highly confident about their ability to cope may sometimes ignore evidence that their efforts were unsuccessful and thus fail to adjust their behavior. A challenge orientation engages us with stressors, but when this tendency is unrelenting, it can lead to physiological exhaustion.[16]

Crucially, though, when these beliefs coalesce to form a flexibility mindset, their possible individual limitations are countered by their synergistic quality. Each part of the mindset enhances the impact of the other two in a way that expands their joint capacity to effectively and appropriately engage us with the task at hand.

Optimism is still a prominent player and frequently functions as the driver of that synergy. When optimism points us to a positive future, for instance, it becomes easier to imagine that we have already solved the challenge. This renders whatever difficult situation we are currently struggling with far more manageable than it would be otherwise. Seeing ourselves in a better future bolsters our confidence that we already have the ability to cope, and that idea can further enhance our confidence that we will be able to manage the challenges we face in the present moment. Optimism can similarly increase our willingness to think of threats in terms of the specific challenges they present. If the future is going to be good, we'd better stop worrying about how threatened we might be feeling and get on with whatever we have to do, whatever the challenge is, that will get us past it.

These influences have an appealing logic about them. But they've also been demonstrated in research using an approach called *path analysis*. One study, for example, compared the relationships between different predictors among disaster survivors and found that the best explanation for good mental health was a "path" that started with optimism and led to increased confidence in coping and then to reduced distress and trauma symptoms. Another path analysis, this time assessing depression in breast cancer patients who had recently undergone chemotherapy, revealed a path that went from optimism to a greater challenge orientation and then to lower depression.[17]

Synergistic pathways also spring from the other direction. Confidence in coping can, for example, enhance our capacity for having a challenge orientation. Again, this has a commonsense logic—the more confident we are in our ability to cope, the more likely it becomes that we will focus on the challenges at hand. But it has also been demonstrated empirically.[18] This pathway was also observed in an experimental study in which participants were given extremely difficult tasks to complete. Many participants initially viewed the tasks as challenges. However, participants in one condition were assigned tasks that were deliberately made to be unsolvable. Not surprisingly, participants confronted with the unsolvable problem gradually stopped thinking of the task as a challenge and reoriented to focusing on how threatening it was. And yet confidence in coping buffered this effect. Participants who were confident in their coping ability at the beginning of the experiment were more likely to persist in viewing the task as a challenge even when they experienced repeated failures. Crucially, these participants were also less likely to feel depressed and discouraged about their performance relative to other participants.[19]

Another experimental study revealed the opposite pathway: in this case, a challenge orientation increased confidence in coping. This study used the so-called cold pressor test, a painful procedure in which participants are instructed to immerse their hands in ice-cold water for as long as possible. Those who perceived the cold pressor task as a challenge, even while their hands were immersed in the icy water, later showed an increase in their sense of personal efficacy, which helped them tolerate the pain for even longer periods of time. Still another study demonstrated that, although optimism often leads to confidence in coping, greater confidence in coping can also reverse the flow and further ramp up optimism. This, too, makes sense. The more we feel we are able to manage ourselves, the better the future looks.[20]

Although it may seem like a bit of a cliché, these research findings clearly demonstrate that a flexibility mindset is more than the sum of its parts. The individual beliefs that contribute to the mindset feed into each other, and by doing so they synergistically expand and reinforce the broader conviction that we will be able to adapt ourselves to the challenges at hand and do whatever is necessary to move forward. The strength of that broader conviction is essential for flexibly responding. We can see this effect in research as well as in firsthand accounts of people faced with serious adversity, as, for example, in the compelling life story of the Mexican artist Frida Kahlo.

Frida

Frida Kahlo is a global icon. Although she was well known during her lifetime—as much for her radical politics and tumultuous marriage with the famous muralist Diego Rivera as for her art—it was not until recently that her image became instantly recognizable. Her fame is well deserved. She was a unique individual and a gifted artist. In her paintings, she found new ways to depict her internal fantasies and struggles, and most of all her lifetime of pain and adversity.

Kahlo's trials began early. At the age of six, she contracted polio. Although she recovered, the illness left its mark on her body. Then, at the age of eighteen, tragedy struck.

She and her boyfriend at the time, Alejandro, were traveling through the streets of Mexico City in a jam-packed wooden bus. The year was 1925. Buses were relatively new to Mexico City and they drew hordes of passengers. The bus drivers could not resist showing off. They drove their new chariots with ostentatious "toreador" bravado.[21]

The bus Kahlo and Alejandro were riding approached an oncoming trolley car. The driver sped up and attempted to skirt in front of the trolley. He badly misjudged the turn, and the trolley plowed into the bus.

Alejandro described what happened next: "Slowly the train pushed the bus. The bus had a strange elasticity. It bent more and more and for a time it did not break. It was a bus with long benches on either side. I remember that at one moment my knees touched the knees of the person sitting opposite me. I was sitting next to Frida. When the bus reached a maximal flexibility, it burst into a thousand pieces, and the train kept moving. It ran over many people."[22]

One of the iron handrails from the bus snapped in two and, in a violent thrust, skewered Kahlo's body, piercing her pelvis and then emerging from the other side. She lay motionless and bloody in the wreckage.

"I picked her up—in those days I was a strong boy—and then I noticed with horror that Frida had a piece of iron in her body. A man said, 'We have to take it out.' He put his knee on Frida's body, and said, 'Let's take it out.' When he pulled it out, Frida screamed so loud that when the ambulance from the Red Cross arrived, her screaming was louder than the siren."[23]

The ambulance transported Kahlo to the nearby Red Cross hospital. Her spinal column was broken in three places. The damage was in the lumbar region, located low in the spinal column, just above the hip. The lumbar vertebrae bear a great deal of the body's weight. This region is also where the spinal cord terminates and forms the two sciatic nerves, which extend the length of the legs all the way to the foot. Together, the lumbar region and the sciatic nerves are crucial for regulating mobility. Unfortunately, they are also infamous as sources of lower back and leg pain. To make matters worse, Kahlo suffered multiple fractures to her foot and pelvis and damage to her internal organs.

The doctors at the hospital were uncertain whether Kahlo would walk again, or for that matter, even survive. They decided the only hope would be to attempt a surgical repair of the damage. When Kahlo regained consciousness, she found herself encased in a full body cast, one of many she would wear throughout her life.

Surprisingly, despite the pain and extent of her injuries, Kahlo recovered quickly, and only one month after the accident she was relocated to the home of her parents, just outside the city. She was still encased in the body cast and still in great pain, but her doctors reasoned that the home atmosphere and fresh air would hasten her recovery.

"My leg hurts so very much . . . and I feel very uncomfortable as you might imagine, but with rest they say that the bone will soon heal and that I'll be able to walk little by little," she wrote in a letter.[24]

The prescription seemed to work. Only three months after the accident, Kahlo was able to walk. She even took a short trip on her own into the heart of the city.

Unfortunately, the miracle turned out to be a mirage, and Kahlo's condition soon deteriorated. It is important to understand that in 1925, little was known about spinal cord injuries or their treatment. Her doctors did not x-ray her spine, largely because it was exorbitantly expensive in those days, and as a result they never adequately assessed the damage to the spinal column. It was only discovered later that the fractured vertebrae had never properly healed.[25]

As time wore on, Kahlo began to suffer from fatigue and nearly debilitating pain. She was frequently nauseous and experienced disturbing periods in which she lost feeling in her legs. Her spinal column was disintegrating. One year after the accident, she found herself back in a full body cast.[26]

Although she eventually improved and was again able to walk, Kahlo's body never fully recovered. She suffered a lifetime of secondary health problems and a seemingly endless array of medical procedures. Her lumbar vertebrae fused, leaving her without the protective cartilage between the bones that would normally cushion impact and movement. Her right foot, broken in multiple places during the accident, also failed to heal properly and provided an additional source of chronic pain. Multiple surgeries didn't help. As she grew older, the pain left her exhausted, as well as vulnerable to a host of other maladies. Eventually her right leg became infected and had to be amputated. A year later, she died. She was only forty-seven.

Was Frida Kahlo resilient? We cannot answer that question with the precision we usually have in our research. We don't have the same kind of data. But amid the abundant biographical materials that we do have—paintings, photos, letters, journal entries, newspaper clippings, reminiscences from friends—Kahlo shines through with undeniable buoyancy. Despite all she endured, nothing remotely like trauma symptoms appears in her letters or diaries. There's no sign of lasting depression, and no apparent anxiety. When her biographer Hayden Herrera examined Kahlo's materials, she was "struck" by "the intensity of her appetite for life—her will not simply to endure but to enjoy."[27] Yes, Kahlo was indefatigable. But she also embodied, in brilliant detail, each of the beliefs that make up the flexibility mindset. Throughout the course of her difficult life, even as a schoolgirl, it was possible to see her burgeoning optimism, her growing sense of confidence in her ability to handle adversity, and her continual readiness to focus on the challenges at hand.[28] It was also possible to see how these beliefs influenced and magnified each other to create in her an appropriate and enduring conviction that she would always manage to adapt to whatever challenges her life threw at her.

When Kahlo contracted polio at the age of six, there was no known cure. Often the disease was fatal. She was bedridden for nine months but eventually recovered, although her right leg was never the same. It was thinner and a bit shorter than her left leg and gave her a slight limp when she walked. To correct the problem, she needed special shoes.

The slimmer right leg embarrassed her. She remembers, "I developed a horrible complex, and to hide my leg I wore thick wool socks up to the knee with bandages underneath."[29]

But despite her embarrassment, or perhaps because of it, Kahlo remained steadfast in her belief that she would find a way to deal with it. Driven by that confidence, she oriented herself toward solving the challenge. When her doctor and her father encouraged her to take up sports as a way to strengthen her body, she didn't hesitate to heed their advice. She played soccer. She swam. She wrestled.

She even took up boxing. And although such activities, especially wrestling and boxing, were viewed as unseemly at the time for a girl from a well-to-do family, that only made Kahlo relish the challenge even more.[30]

It was at this time that she also discovered with great joy that she had an aptitude for fantasy and could use that skill to help her cope with her tribulations.

"This was during the period when I had my imaginary friend," she later told an interviewer. "I would look out of the small glass panes of the window and fill them with steam. Then, I would draw a little window and go out through it. Opposite our house, there was a milk store that was named Pinźon, and I would travel from the little window through the 'o' in Pinźon, and from there to the center of the earth, where I had my friend, and we would dance and play. If I was called at that moment, I would go behind a tree and hide, and I would laugh, very happy." She added, "Other times, I sat on the small steps that faced the stone patio. There was an oven for baking bread in front of the kitchen, and I would make believe that I saw little boys and girls dressed in pink coming out of the oven. They would come in groups and then disappear. It gave me so much pleasure."[31]

Years later, when she relapsed for the first time after the spinal cord injury, Kahlo had to remain bedridden and immobilized for much longer periods of time. That did not come readily to such a restless and inquisitive spirit. Unlike her recovery from polio, which was aided by physical activity, convalescence after the spinal cord injury required stillness. It would have been easy to let idleness overwhelm her, to let herself fall into a deep depression. But her optimism and confidence helped her orient toward this new challenge, and that combination in turn led her to a resoundingly flexible solution, one she would rely on for the rest of her life. She took up painting.

"I was bored as hell in bed with a plaster cast . . . so I decided to do something. I stole from my father some oil paints, and my mother ordered for me a special easel because I couldn't sit . . . and I started to paint."[32]

She painted anything she could see. Her foot. Her body casts. Friends who visited. And eventually, after her family had a mirror suspended above her bed so that she could see her own reflection, she painted herself.

Finding such a perfect solution to her dilemma boosted Kahlo's sense of coping efficacy and further amplified her already irrepressible optimism, much to the chagrin of her doctors, whom Kahlo regularly frustrated by disregarding their orders "to live quietly and restfully."[33] But her urgency to overcome her physical limitations was palpable.

When her injuries finally healed, Kahlo quickly resumed her previous energetic lifestyle. Although she did not return to school, she renewed connections with many of the same circle of friends. She attended parties, political rallies, and cultural events.

It was around this time that Diego Rivera became a fixture in her life. Already a world-renowned painter, Rivera had been living in Paris and had only recently returned to Mexico City to paint murals. He had actually met Kahlo briefly several years earlier, when as a schoolgirl she had asked for permission to watch him paint. Even then, Rivera remembered, "she had an unusual dignity and self-assurance, and there was a strange fire in her eyes." Later, after she had begun to paint seriously, Kahlo boldly approached Rivera again, this time bringing along three of her own paintings to show him. Her brash spirit struck Rivera. He felt "moved by admiration" for her, and a week later he visited the Kahlo home to see the rest of her work. Recalling the moment in his autobiography, he wrote, "I did not know it then but Frida had already become the most important fact in my life. And she would continue to be, up to the moment she died, twenty-seven years later."[34]

Rivera and Kahlo soon began spending a great deal of time to-gether. One day, Kahlo's father took Rivera aside, as Rivera reported in his autobiography:

> "I see you are interested in my daughter, eh?" he said.
> "Yes," I replied, "otherwise I would not be coming all the way out to Coyoacán to see her."
> "She is a devil," he said.
> "I know it."
> "Well, I've warned you," he said, and he left.[35]

But Kahlo's bold and mischievous nature was precisely what ap-pealed most to Rivera. In a very short time, they married. It was only four years after Kahlo's spinal cord injury.

They made for a striking couple. Rivera was a large man, over six feet tall and rotund. Kahlo was small and slender, with intense features. Together, they dwelled at the epicenter of a cultural and political whirlwind and quickly became media darlings, dubbed "the elephant and the dove." They were photographed frequently in the company of their celebrated friends, including writers, artists, and political figures.[36]

Kahlo and Rivera's life together was active and rich and full. They protested in the streets. They traveled. They entertained. They were tender with each other. They were passionate, and sometimes their relationship was tumultuous. They fought, and frequently, they were unfaithful. Rivera in particular was renowned for his infidelities, but Kahlo, too, had affairs, most famously with the exiled Russian revo-lutionary Leon Trotsky and the sculptor Isamu Noguchi.

In her later years, Kahlo found ways to reconcile these divergent aspects of her life. But her body increasingly failed her. Gradually her life evolved into a constant struggle with pain and exhaustion.

In 1950, at the age of forty-three, she recorded in her journal, "I have been sick for one year now. Seven operations on my spinal column . . . I don't know if I will be able to walk again soon. I have a plaster corset. Even though it is a frightful nuisance, it helps my spine. I don't feel any pain. Only this bloody tiredness, and naturally quite often, despair."[37]

At several points in her life, Kahlo contemplated suicide, not from depression but rather "out of desperation" over the relentless physical pain.[38]

"If I felt better, health-wise, one could say that I am happy," she admitted.[39] "I am not sick. I am broken. But I am happy to be alive as long as I can paint."[40]

The Red Boots

Even as her body failed her, Kahlo's flexibility mindset continually fostered an ability to counter the challenges of her life. She confidently invented novel ways to express herself, which provided her and others with obvious pleasure. They also served as flexible solutions to help her endure, and sometimes mask, her ongoing difficulties.

The writer Carlos Fuentes recalls a striking encounter with Kahlo at an opera:

> I was in the Palace of Fine Arts of Mexico and the opera that night was Wagner. The overture was being played and suddenly a noise invaded the theater that silenced the orchestra. We all looked up to the balcony and saw the magnificent, the regal entrance of Frida Kahlo. With all these jewels on. The necklaces. The rings. The bracelets. The things in her hair. It all jangled in such a way like it was a cathedral gone mad, with all the bells jangling at the same time, made to distract from the weakness of her body, the fact that it was a crippled body, a dying body, always. And she gave it life through the jewels and the dresses and the whole . . . her own opera! There was Wagner on the stage, but there was Frida Kahlo on the balcony. And that night at least she was stronger than Wagner, to be sure.[41]

Her knack for embracing challenges reinforced her optimism, or perhaps it might be fairer to say that it staved off a looming pessimism. For the pain was growing more difficult over time. But this only became, for Kahlo, the ultimate challenge. She loved to defy expectations about her disability.

"I knew Frida well during an eight-month period," wrote Noguchi. "We went dancing all the time. Frida loved to dance. That was her passion, you know, everything that she couldn't do she loved to do. It made her absolutely furious to be unable to do things."[42]

One of the most difficult periods in Kahlo's life occurred when she learned that her leg was to be amputated. Just prior to the surgery, a group of friends visited her. Seeing their concern, Kahlo "tried to cheer them up with stories and jokes." One friend, the art historian Antonio Rodriguez, remarked, "We were almost in tears seeing this marvelous, beautiful and optimistic woman, and knowing they were going to amputate her leg."[43]

The amputation was hard on her. Life is not easy for people with disabilities, and the world was not nearly as accommodating to disability in Kahlo's time as it is now. For someone who needed excitement and activity as much as Kahlo, the loss of a leg was nothing short of an affront. And after the surgery, for a brief period, she succumbed. She became demoralized and depressed. She spoke of suicide. But it didn't last long.

Kahlo was especially upset by the wooden prosthetic leg she had been given. Aesthetically it was offensive to her. She thought it ugly, and she had a difficult time walking with it. But by this point in her long journey she was nearly indelibly optimistic and soon that optimism roared back. As it did, Kahlo shifted her focus and reoriented herself toward yet another new challenge. When her enduring confidence kicked in, she knew she would find a solution. And she did, a wonderfully inventive one. She had a special pair of high-heeled boots made in striking red leather and adorned with gold silk embroidery and tiny bells. The boots not only concealed the prosthesis, but they equaled her brilliantly colorful wardrobe while at the same time allowing her the greater mobility she craved. When she first tried them on, she was so pleased that she felt she would "dance her joy": "And she twirled in front of friends to show off her new freedom of movement," as one friend described it. The writer Carlota Tibon recalled sometime later that Kahlo had danced an almost gymnastic *jarabe tapatío* (Mexican hat dance) for her. Bursting with pride, she had said, "These marvelous legs! And how well they work for me!"[44]

The success again fortified Kahlo's confidence that she would always be able to meet the challenges of her demanding life head-on and that she would continue to thrive. Her satisfaction was not misplaced. The red boots were truly a work of art in their own right. They have survived to this day and can be viewed in the Frida Kahlo Museum in Mexico City.[45] Even in photographs, the boots evoke a certain awe. Created over seventy years ago, they were ahead of their time and look as beautiful as they must have the day she first wore them.

Reinvention

Above all else, Kahlo's flexibility mindset allowed her to channel her struggles into her paintings. In her extraordinary work, she found the ultimate solution to the ultimate challenge.

Although relatively unacknowledged as a serious artist until late in her life, Kahlo's paintings became her enduring legacy. They are luminous and compelling, crafted in a novel style of her own discovery, a dreamlike realism that mixes narrative folk elements, figures, symbols, animals, and even medical equipment. The paintings were sometimes mischievous, sometimes strikingly macabre. But for Kahlo they became an indispensable solution, a way for her to live with the difficulties she had no choice but to endure.

Kahlo herself once said, "As the accident changed my path, many things prevented me from fulfilling the desires which everyone considers normal, and to me nothing seemed more normal than to paint what had not been fulfilled."[46]

Flexibility is essentially a process of transformation and reinvention. Kahlo's paintings allowed her to reinvent herself each time her body failed her. In this way they stand as a stunning example of how flexibility can function in the struggle to overcome adversity. As one of her close friends, the photographer Lola Álvarez Bravo, observed, "Frida is the only painter who gave birth to herself."[47] And, in fact, several of Kahlo's paintings delved deeply into the symbolism of birth.

During a visit to the United States, where Rivera had been commissioned to create several murals, Kahlo became pregnant. Despite her physical limitations, she desperately wished for a child. Her doctors had given her hope that a successful birth might be possible by cesarean section. One night, when they were visiting Detroit, where Diego was working on a mural, she began to bleed profusely. She was rushed to the hospital. The baby could not be saved, and Kahlo nearly succumbed as well. She had lost a great deal of blood and needed to remain in the hospital for thirteen days to get her strength back. Initially she was distraught and deeply grieved.

Once again, she reoriented herself to the challenge. And painting once again provided the solution that saved her.

As her biographer Hayden Herrera described it, "Five days after her miscarriage, she took up a pencil and drew a bust-length self-portrait. In it she wears a kimono and a hair net, and her face is swollen with tears. And even in the midst of misery she could find laughter."[48]

Kahlo wanted desperately to draw her lost child. She requested medical books but the hospital refused. They told her the hospital did not allow patients to have such books because they believed they would be too upsetting for them.

"Frida was furious," wrote Herrera. "But Diego interceded, telling the doctor, 'You are not dealing with an average person. Frida will do something with it. She will do artwork.'"[49]

Eventually Rivera obtained the medical books himself and brought them to Kahlo. She made pencil studies of a fetus and several other drawings related to her miscarriage. Later that same year she created two more elaborate paintings on the same theme. In one, *Henry Ford Hospital*, she depicted herself naked and bleeding on a hospital bed, as if suspended in space, with the city of Detroit in the background. She is tethered to six blood-red tubes, each connected to a symbolic object: a fetus, a womb, a snail, an orchid (given to her by Rivera), a pelvis, and a mechanical medical device. The other painting, titled *My Birth*, depicts Kahlo's own birth. The painting shows a female torso on a bed with Kahlo's head appearing from the womb.

Although Kahlo also painted and sketched more conventional portraits of friends and family, her exceedingly original self-portraits are without a doubt her most accomplished works. In these paintings, she looks directly into the viewer's eyes with an arresting gaze. Her mouth is closed, but the intensity of her scrutiny seems to speak an elaborate story. Many of the self-portraits are strikingly beautiful. Some are mystical, some profoundly disquieting. She often filled them with symbolic objects—sometimes with monkeys or birds, often with elements of her infirmities. One of her most famous self-portraits, *The Broken Column*, is stark, barren, surreal, almost medieval. Kahlo depicts herself, seminude and harnessed in the medical brace she was at that time forced to wear, as if being tortured. She stands in a barren landscape. Nails have been driven into her body. Tears flow from her eyes. Her torso is split down the middle from her chin to her abdomen, revealing a rigid steel shaft in place of the spinal cord. Her expression is plaintive and passionless.

But the intensity of Kahlo's self-portraits belies the fact that they renewed her and fed her. Each portrait expressed a different aspect of her struggle. By depicting her pain, her suffering, love, curiosity, and intrigue, the paintings allowed her to live with renewed confidence and optimism. Each of these paintings seems to boldly say, "This is my life. This is my challenge. Look what I have done with it."

It is difficult to ignore these paintings. Like the idea of resilience itself, they are at once obvious and elusive. Near the end of her life, when she had to face the pending amputation of her leg, Kahlo painted a picture in her journal of two dismembered feet. The feet are freestanding, like fragments of a Roman statue, but with severed veins graphically rising out of the top. The page is tinted by a wash of bloodred paint. Strangely, the overall impression is not gruesome. A more apt descriptor would be "mischievous." Once again, we see Kahlo's optimism, her indefatigable self-confidence, and her willing embrace of her life challenges, all rolled into the single synergistic conviction that whatever befell her, she would always find a way to thrive. At the bottom of the page, impishly, she wrote, "Feet, what do I need them for if I have wings to fly."[50]

More Than a Mindset

There is no denying that Frida Kahlo was a compelling individual. Maren, in her own way, is equally compelling. I chose their stories for this book in part because they so perfectly illustrate how the belief system underpinning a flexibility mindset—optimism, confidence in coping, and a challenge orientation—put us in the right frame of mind for finding adaptive solutions. But there is a risk in using stories of such remarkable individuals: they can seem to imply that the flexibility mindset is only for exceptional people, that somehow it is preordained for them, but well out of reach for most "normal" people. Fortunately, this is not the case. Most people are resilient, and most people are reasonably flexible. Although some are more likely than others to gravitate toward this way of thinking, the beliefs that go into a flexibility mindset can be cultivated, and they can be utilized at any time by anyone willing to try.

There is another risk, though, in relying on stories from such compelling individuals. Their impressive accomplishments can easily lead to the false assumption that a flexibility mindset is all we need—that once we have cultivated a conviction in our ability to adapt, for the most part the job is done. The stories and the research both demonstrate clearly how indispensable that conviction can be. But we still need to take the next step. We still need to find a way to adjust ourselves to meet the challenges we face. We've seen plenty of examples of flexible solutions—from Maren and Frida Kahlo, especially—but we haven't yet seen exactly how they came to those solutions. For that we need to look at the second component, or rather, set of components, of the flexibility process.

PART IV

Nuts and Bolts

CHAPTER 7

The Flexibility Sequence

You've heard the refrain now many times. Once we are engaged and motivated, we must next somehow determine the right behavior for the right situation at the right time. Assuming this all makes sense—and I will devote the next few chapters to convincing you that it does—then undoubtedly someone must have hit on the idea before. As it turns out, the ancient Greeks knew about flexibility, or at least as far as I can tell they did. I am not a scholar of the classics. But this passage from Aristotle's seminal work on ethics seems to fit the bill: "Anybody can become angry—that is easy. . . . [B]ut to be angry with . . . the right person, and to the right amount, and at the right time, and for the right purpose, and in the right way. That . . . is not easy."[1]

Aristotle was right. Flexibility is not easy, especially when we are confronted with the chaos and intensity of traumatic stress. Of course, there is always the option of doing nothing. Passively waiting it out. Simply managing as best we can without engaging. The aphorism "Time heals all wounds" does have some truth to it. But time is usually in no hurry, and simply waiting for the pain to go away can be exhausting, if not debilitating. It is far less anguishing, and more effective, to face our foreboding head-on and do whatever we need to in order to move forward.

Again, this is not a new idea. This time it is the Roman philosopher Seneca who considered the topic, when he advised, "We must make ourselves flexible. . . . [W]e should make the transition to the state that chance has brought us to without dreading a change either in our purpose or our condition. For stubbornness, from which Fortune often forces some concession, must involve anxiety and wretchedness."[2]

Luckily, the process by which we do this, by which we "make ourselves flexible," is not a blind stab in the dark. It is an orderly process, and, in fact, a growing body of research has begun to illuminate the nature of that orderly process. I've alluded to this research already in our discussion of the flexibility sequence. Now we can take a closer look at what that sequence entails.

The first step in the sequence is *context sensitivity*. We can't respond effectively to a situation if we don't know what we are responding to. When we are sensitized to the situational context, we are able to decode the cues, determine what is happening to us, and figure out what to do about it. Once we have this answer—once we know what we need to do—we slide naturally into the next step, called *repertoire*. Here we work out not only what we need to do, but what we are able to do, and what we are able to do depends on the kinds of tools we have at our disposal, our repertoire. We then come to the third and final step, *feedback monitoring*. At this point, we engage in an underappreciated but absolutely essential correction process. Even the most skilled person makes mistakes. It is not uncommon, actually, to judge incorrectly and choose an ineffective strategy, a strategy that is not quite as effective as we'd hoped. The feedback monitoring step is where we have a chance to adjust or change that response.

The two broad components of the flexibility process, the flexibility mindset and the flexibility sequence, work in concert in ways that sometimes blur the distinction between them. To better highlight the unique steps of the flexibility sequence, and how they hinge on, but also extend beyond, the flexibility mindset, we'll take some time to explore the entire flexibility process as it unfolds in the aftermath of a nasty situation that befell a fellow named Paul.

Paul

Paul was in a good mood. It had been a long day. But a good day. And after work, he decided to stop by the apartment of two old friends, Mark and Laura. Paul had known Mark and Laura for years. They didn't know he was coming, and he knew it probably wasn't the best time to visit. Mark and Laura had two young children and most likely they would be in the process of preparing the evening meal. But Paul didn't intend to stay long. Just a quick hello.

Luckily, Mark and Laura's children happened to be spending the night with Laura's mother. Their evening was free and they were delighted to see Paul. Together they shared a few drinks, then moved on to a long and pleasant dinner.

It was late when Paul finally ambled home. He initially planned to grab a cab, but, since the evening had been so pleasant, he decided to walk. It had rained earlier. Chicago was always more pleasant after a rain. "Cleaner and fresher," Paul thought. "Lights reflecting off the pavement were beautiful."

As he walked, his thoughts drifted back to the conversations he'd had with his friends. Laura had told a funny but sad story about their son. It touched Paul. He would have liked to have had children of his own. That was unlikely, and he knew it. He had dated a lot of women, but for one reason or another, the relationships never worked out. He did have a girlfriend now. It was going well, but

171

she was probably past her childbearing years, and, in any case, she'd made it clear she wasn't interested in having children.

Paul was still mulling all this over when he turned and walked along a street bordering a park. He had only walked a few blocks when he felt his phone vibrating in his pocket. It was a text from Mark. "THX for dropping by. Sooooo GR8 to CU." Then another: "but dude you left your bag." Paul stopped in his tracks. Should he go back? There were papers in the bag he would need tomorrow, at work. It was an unfortunate turn of events. It had been such a nice evening. He thought for a moment and then continued walking. He texted Mark, "I'll come by in the am? When u guys up???," and then upon reflection added, "Oh wait. Sorry. UR kids away."

Paul waited for Mark's response, his phone glowing in the dark, and then he turned and entered the park.

"I cut through the park at night. It was no big deal," Paul remembered. "Back when I first moved here, then, that was like a while ago now, it was way too dangerous. But it's different. Now it's pretty safe. I don't always feel like, you know, nothing can happen. I know stuff happens. But, generally, it's safe."

Paul remembered seeing other people walking in the distance. To him, this meant it was safe. People were out.

He texted Mark again. "Is it ok, coming by in the morning??"

About thirty seconds later, Mark responded, "sure tomorrow. good. i'll be home."

Paul texted back, "thanks. Don't go pawing my stuff. Big boy papers in there."

Mark responded, "ORLY. THX for idea."

"Ha," Paul said out loud, grinning. He began to text a response. "u r . . ."

Something struck his head, hard and sharp. He fell forward, confused. As he began turning to look behind him, something else slammed him from the right side.

"It knocked the wind out of me. Man, I went right down."

Crouching on the pavement, Paul could see several figures jostling around him.

"It was dark. You know, I couldn't see anything. But I saw enough, to know, it was bad."

He tried to speak.

Then a forceful kick to his side.

"I couldn't breathe. I was like trying to say, you know, something to stop it. I don't know exactly what. I must have said something like, 'Wait, please. Don't hurt me. I'll give you whatever you want.' I don't really remember but based on what happened, that's what I must have said.

"I don't think I actually got the words out. I couldn't breathe. It was just going really fast."

Another blow flattened him.

Paul felt the rough texture of the pavement scraping against his face. He tried to speak.

"I remember this voice. I remember it, you know like a high-pitched, a deliberate high pitch, like a falsetto, mocking me. Imitating me, like 'Pleeeese, don't hurt me,' in this high falsetto. It sickens me even now to remember it. You know it was like some torture thing."

Another kick to the side. His body screamed with pain.

Paul's mind was racing.

Then something hard struck him in the side of the face.

"I don't remember much more. I wanted to disappear. I just, I didn't want to exist there, you know, in that moment. But I do. The ringing. I remember the ringing. My head felt like a rock, like a solid piece of, I don't know, concrete or something, and my ears were ringing. Then, I don't know. It got quiet. I think I must have passed out."

•

PAUL STRUGGLED TO open his eyes. He was unsure where he was or how long he had been there. He could hear voices in the distance.

He tried to track them as best he could. They faded and disappeared. He drifted off.

He opened his eyes again. He remembered thinking that some time must have passed.

"I could sort of tell. The light had changed."

He tried to call out. Uncertainty overwhelmed him.

"I opened my mouth, but it was like, nothing. No sound. I was mute. No sound came out."

Sometime later—he wasn't sure how much later—he heard a dog. He became more alert, aware that he was on the ground.

He rolled over.

"My shirt was soaking wet. I didn't know. Was I in a puddle or what, maybe blood. I remember I was scared right then. Really scared."

He called out but heard nothing.

He wrenched his body upward. Pain flashed through his shoulder and side. His head was pounding. He felt nauseous.

Eventually, he managed to stand up. He touched his face and winced. He could feel caked blood.

He staggered toward the lights, several blocks away, and felt his pockets. His phone and wallet were gone.

"It was still dark. I had no idea what time it was. But I could more or less figure out where I was. I knew there was a hospital. I knew where the hospital was. I could walk."

He looked around anxiously. Nobody in sight.

He was bloody and frightened and began walking.

"It really hurt to move. I started, you know, walking like a guy in a zombie movie. But I had this horrible feeling, like someone, these guys, were still there, somewhere, you know, watching and waiting for me. They were going to get me again. The same guys.

"I got to the end of the park. Nothing happened. Nobody. I didn't see anyone. I crossed the street, turning around, you know, as

I walked, like waking in a kind of circle. I was trying to see if anyone was coming."

He saw no one.

He kept going, more steadily now. A block away from the park, his thoughts calmed a little. He reached up and touched his head and face. Definitely swollen and bloody, but maybe not too bad. The hospital wasn't far. He would be safe once he got there. He could get himself patched up.

The taunts of his attackers popped back into his consciousness.

"I kept hearing the sound of that voice in my head, the falsetto voice."

Paul makes a mocking face and imitates the voice: "Pleeeese, don't hurt me. Pleeese. Oh pleeease, don't hurt me."

He shudders.

"I still remember it, right now, perfectly. It just cuts me, you know, right through me.

"That night, I felt as bad as I've ever felt. Small, just really small, pitiful. You know, totally ashamed. I was blaming myself. For walking through the park. I was thinking it was my fault for acting that way, for being such, I don't know, a coward."

•

PAUL'S INJURIES WERE not as serious as he had feared. He needed stitches on his forehead, above the right eye. His face was scraped and he was badly bruised. But no broken bones. No concussion. The neurologist gave him a list of possible symptoms to look out for, but otherwise his prognosis was okay.

By the time Paul finally reached his apartment, the sun was coming up. He was frazzled. But before he could try to get some sleep, there were a few urgent matters to attend to. First, he went online and notified his bank and canceled his credit cards. Then he looked into replacing his driver's license. These were annoying tasks but also distracting and strangely comforting. His accounts hadn't been breached. That was good. He felt at least some sense of control again.

He searched online for his phone. Nothing. His attackers had probably already realized it was useless and destroyed it. This was good, too, but thinking about his phone brought back the painful memories. He imagined his attackers laughing as they smashed it against a rock.

"I tried to clear my mind. I knew that I should be letting people know what happened. But you . . . The idea, it just mortified me."

The best he could manage was to email his job to say he'd be taking a sick day. Then he emailed Mark to let him know he wouldn't be coming over after all, but didn't say why. He emailed Carrie, his girlfriend, to explain that she might not have been able to reach him but, again, he didn't mention the mugging. He said only that he'd lost his phone.

"My head was kind of spinning. I felt kind of nauseous."

"I couldn't get it out of my head. I was doing the replay. Seeing it all again. I kept thinking about those guys, the way I acted. I had this image of how they must have seen me. The guys that attacked me, you know, in their eyes. There I was, on the ground. Scared. Pleading. I must have looked pitiful, whimpering and pleading, 'Don't hurt me.'"

He wanted nothing more than to turn it all off. But how?

Context Sensitivity

The first step in the flexibility sequence, *context sensitivity*, is a vital skill, possibly the most vital skill of the sequence, because it helps us determine what is happening at a particular moment and how we might best respond. We've already gotten a sense of this step with the components of the flexibility mindset: optimism, confidence in coping, and challenge orientation, which work together to motivate us and help us engage with the situational demands before us.

Context sensitivity builds on this process by focusing much more specifically on the details, on the particular contextual nuances and demands we face. In essence, in this step we ask ourselves, "What is happening to me?" "What is the problem?" and "What do I need to do to get past it?"

Although most people are reasonably sensitive to context, there is, as with any ability, variation. Oddly, though, even when people are capable of these kinds of contextual evaluations, they often fail to give them much thought. They may feel troubled, for example, or uneasy or anxious, but not sure why. Sometimes simply asking the question "What is bothering me?" can help a person focus more closely on what exactly is actually happening. But even when people ask themselves this kind of question, they still have to be able to read the cues. And clearly, some people have deficits in this skill. In other words, some people are relatively context insensitive.

Research has shown that context-insensitive people tend to struggle more psychologically and often to experience poorer mental health overall.[3] My own research explored this issue by asking people to read descriptions of various hypothetical situations—for example, being stuck in an elevator or returning home after a vacation to find that your home has been robbed—and then to evaluate each situation for different types of situational cues (such as the level of threat the situation represented, how urgently a response might be needed, and the degree of control they would have over it).[4] We found that people varied in their ability to evaluate the cues. For example, people who were depressed or anxious tended to have a harder time determining when a situation was or was not threatening, and therefore when it required an urgent response. These correlations are tricky to interpret. There are myriad reasons why a person might develop psychological problems, and even depressed people are sometimes able to read contextual cues. In fact, in one study we found that depressed people with intact context-sensitivity skills were more likely to improve over time than those with only minimal context sensitivity. The former were more likely to show a recovery trajectory, while the latter were more likely to experience depression for an extended period of time.[5]

A key aspect of context sensitivity is the ability to detect changes in contextual cues.[6] This skill was nicely demonstrated by a team led by my colleague Einat Levy-Gigi using a simple computer game.[7] The game presented people with a series of boxes, one box at a time. Each box was a different color and had a picture of a common object on it. For example, a picture of a television might appear on a green box, while a picture of a hat might appear on a yellow box, and so on. Each time players saw a box, they had to decide whether to open it or not. If they opened the box and there was money inside, they received points. If they opened the box and there was a bomb inside, they lost points. Gradually, players learned which combinations of box colors and objects they should open and which combinations they should not open. Critically, once the players got good at the game, new variations were introduced. Without any notification, the game would begin to present new pairings of colored boxes and objects along with the original pairings of colored boxes and objects. For example, the television on a green box that had earned points still earned points, but now a television appearing on a red box resulted in the loss of points. The only way to come out ahead was to be sensitive to these subtle changes in the contextual cues.

Some of the most interesting findings emerged when a box color that originally produced a negative outcome later might also produce a positive outcome. For example, a hat on a blue box originally meant there would be a bomb in the box while later in the game a car on a blue box meant there would be money inside. The study showed that the ability to track when a box that was originally negative could also later be positive was predicted by the size of the player's hippocampus. This was an impressive finding. The hippocampus is a crucial brain structure involved in the perception, memory, and understanding of context. Einat and her colleagues also showed that people with chronic PTSD symptoms had a particularly difficult time learning this same negative-to-positive context change. This also makes perfect sense, because one of the hallmarks of chronic PTSD symptoms is the tendency to feel that the original traumatic situation is still occurring even in contexts that are generally safe or benign.

How we respond to situations also depends on the broader contexts of our lives and life goals.[8] We saw this kind of interplay when Frida Kahlo struggled with her new prosthesis following the amputation of her leg. She hated the prosthesis. It impeded her movement and she thought it horribly unattractive. This frustrated her and made her sad. If that was all that troubled her, she probably would have tried to find ways to reduce her emotional pain. But the prosthesis went beyond an immediate threat because it also violated her larger life goals: maintaining mobility, dressing colorfully and expressively, and, above all, dancing. By asking herself what the situation demanded in terms of this larger, goal-driven context, she was able to find a creative way to satisfy both her immediate and longer-term challenges.

Paul rarely thought about his long-term goals. When pressed, he would say he liked his job and was striving to advance his career. He also saw himself as a social person who valued his friendships. He'd been working long hours of late, but he had been making efforts to see his friends more often. He also hoped for a stable, long-term relationship. Although his success in this area had not been so good, he seemed to be on the right track in his relationship with Carrie. She was adamant about not wanting children, which was a sore spot for him, but they got along well, and Paul hoped the relationship would stick.

•

THE IMMEDIATE THREAT of a potentially traumatic event often shifts all other goals to the background. The first few days after the mugging, whatever Paul might have thought about his longer-term goals was lost in the haze of traumatic stress. He knew he should contact his friends and colleagues to let them know about the assault. But he couldn't bring himself to tell anyone: not his colleagues at work, not his friends, not even Carrie. Because his face was obviously bruised, with stitches, this meant he could not see anybody, either. He did manage to have a new phone delivered to his apartment, but couldn't bring himself to set it up. Carrie emailed a few times about that. "A tech guy like you, and you haven't set up your phone? What's up with that?" She tried to make plans to see him. Paul stalled with excuses. He knew the tactic was wearing thin.

"The problem was that I felt awful."

Paul was anxious. He felt ashamed. He was sleeping poorly. He'd doze off only to wake in a panic from strange dreams. He knew he should get out of the apartment, but even the thought of going outside made him feel exposed. What if he encountered his attackers? He didn't actually know what they looked like, or at least he had no real memory of their appearance. But he worried they might recognize him. They could be watching him without his knowing it and secretly taunt him, or worse, grab him and assault him all over again.

The third night after his assault, Paul sat for some time staring out his window. Although it was dark, as usual there were plenty of people out and about. Some were busily hurrying off to who knows where. Others were strolling casually. It pained Paul to remember that he used to be one of those people, simply going about his business.

As he imagined himself out on the street, safe and unworried, his mind turned. He began to reflect on his situation. It occurred to him that if he had felt that way before, eventually the feeling would return. The world would right itself. For the first time in days, he felt a glimmer of hope. He actually began to feel optimistic.

If I could have asked Paul, in that moment, if he had a flexibility mindset, he would have stared at me blankly. But whether he knew it or not, reflecting on his life as he gazed out the window, he was able to muster enough of a mindset to motivate himself and engage with his troubles.

The sensation was fleeting. Paul tried to hold on to it. He tried to convince himself.

"C'mon Paul," he said out loud. "Get a grip. You can get past this. You're a smart guy. You can figure it out."

He was boosting his confidence and orienting himself to the challenge.

It was only a subtle shift in attitude, but it was enough to edge Paul more fully into the conviction that he could figure it out.

As he spoke the words out loud—"You can figure it out"— the fog in his brain seemed to lift. The world around him literally seemed to come into sharper focus, and he became increasingly sensitized to contextual cues.

"You know, looking at the neighborhood like that, out the window, I saw. It's great. It's a great neighborhood. It's alive. It's active. I mean, sure, bad stuff happens. There is always something like that, crime. It's the big city. But on the whole, the neighborhood, it's good. It's pretty safe, as long as I've lived here. I used to feel safe. Why shouldn't I be able to feel that way again?"

It was a simple truth, but for Paul it was like an epiphany, and it sparked a cascade of new insights.

"I was just kind of looking out the window and it just hit me. These guys, the guys who attacked me, I had no idea who they were. They didn't know me. They probably didn't even live in this neighborhood. And, you know, odds are if they saw me, they wouldn't recognize me. I mean it was dark. I could pass them on the street, and they wouldn't even know it was me. And probably, they could care less. They were just out to rob someone. I happened to come along, staring at my phone. I was in the wrong place. The wrong place at the wrong time.

"At that moment, everything just kind of simplified. I had cooked up this whole story. These guys were going to come back, look for me, get me again. But they got what they wanted. I had no idea what they did next. Whatever. Probably nothing. They probably never gave me another thought."

Paul began to work it out. First, he would focus on gaining some control over the horrible thoughts and feelings he was having. He knew his neighborhood was safe, logically. He wanted to feel that way again, but he didn't really believe it yet. He was still plagued by cringing doubt. He would have to find a way to shed that doubt, at least long enough to take a step forward. Then, once he could do that, he would make himself get back out there. He would rejoin the world. He knew that wasn't going to be easy, and it wasn't clear yet exactly how he was going to do it. But at least now he knew what he had to do.

Repertoire

The ability to read the cues of a demanding situation is a big piece of the flexibility sequence. Once that piece is in place, the next step in the sequence, repertoire, takes over. Here we take stock of the tools we have in our tool box, our response repertoire. The question changes from "What do I need to do?" to "What am I *able* to do?"

As we saw, most people read the situational cues with at least some basic proficiency, though some people are more context sensitive than others. The same is true for the response repertoire. Take, for example, coping and emotion regulation strategies. Most people have the basic skills for coping and regulating their emotions. But some people are simply better at these skills than others, and have more coping and emotion regulation tools at their disposal. In other words, they have a larger strategy *repertoire*.

It is important to note, though, that responding effectively requires more than simply using a lot of strategies. Indeed, the range of possible strategies is practically limitless.[9] Some of the most common, as I mentioned a few chapters back, are expressing and suppressing emotion, distracting ourselves, reappraising or changing the meaning of an event, strategizing and planning ways to solve the problem, and trying to modify the situation itself. Yet studies have shown that the most frequently used strategies are not always the most successful strategies.[10] Depending on the particulars of a specific challenge, myriad others might prove useful: engaging in wishful thinking or passive acceptance, doing nothing, lying to oneself, escaping or leaving, seeking out information, getting drunk or using drugs, complaining, seeking out the companionship of other people, engaging in self-pity, trying to find comfort in food or sex, avoiding people, asking for help, blaming someone, seeking a release through exercise, trying to feel better through humor or amusements, or just about anything else a person might think to try. Some of these behaviors are undeniably healthy, while others are less so, and some, as you have probably noticed, would fall into the "ugly coping" category. The key point is that the more strategies we are able to engage in effectively, even if we use them only sparingly, the more options we have for meeting the demands of a specific situation.

Back when I first began to explore strategy repertoire, I designed an experiment to measure the ability to effectively use two opposing strategies, emotional expression and emotional suppression. Participants in this experiment viewed photos on a computer—some highly disturbing, some pleasant—and had to rate their emotional reactions to the photos. Once they got used to doing this, they were asked to continue viewing and rating the photos, except now, they were told, another participant in an adjacent room would be watching them from a monitor and trying to guess their emotional reactions. They also learned that different instructions about expressing emotion would appear at different times on the computer. Sometimes the instructions would say to express whatever emotion they felt as fully as possible, so that the observer in the adjacent room could more easily guess what they were feeling. This was the *expression condition*. Other times they would be asked to conceal any emotions they felt, so that the person in the adjacent room would *not* be able to guess what they were feeling. This was the *suppression condition*. There was also a *control condition*, in which participants were told that the camera had been temporarily turned off, and that during this time the observer would not be able to see them. In this case, they should simply view the photos as they would normally. I included the control condition because people differ in how expressive they are naturally, and this allowed me to measure how able they were to show more or less emotion relative to their normal levels.

The experiment worked as I predicted. We hadn't asked participants to vary how they felt while watching the photos, and, as expected, they reported about the same level of emotion across all the conditions. But we did ask them to vary how much emotion they showed, and, on average, we found they could do this. I called this skill *expressive flexibility*. Not surprisingly, we observed variations in this skill. Some people were better at expressing and suppressing emotion than others.[11]

So is it useful to have expressive flexibility in one's repertoire? Does it help people manage traumatic stress? As I was contemplating how to answer this question, fate and the 9/11 attacks intervened. I had originally developed the expressive flexibility task over the summer of 2001. The plan was to include it in a long-term study of mental health among undergraduates. We had just begun the study when it had to be sidelined because of the attacks. When we resumed, weeks later, we realized we were now conducting a trauma study. And the results clearly suggested that expressive flexibility, as measured following 9/11, did help the students cope with traumatic stress. Those who were more expressively flexible had better mental health when we assessed them again two years later. These results also showed that being good at just one of the strategies, expression or suppression, but not both, was not protective. In other words, true to the repertoire concept, the strategies themselves were not as important as the ability to engage in either strategy as needed.[12]

These findings raised an intriguing question: If expressive flexibility helps people cope with traumatic stress, do they know that they have this ability? You might remember the research we discussed earlier showing that most people aren't actually very aware of the coping strategies they used. Was there any reason to think the story would be different if we asked people about the strategies they were good at? My hunch was that the answer would be yes. Knowing what we are good at is a different kind of self-knowledge than knowing how often we do it. When we try to remember how often we do something, we have to remember specific events and then estimate the frequency. But to know whether or not we are good at something requires only that we know we have done it well. And when we tested this idea directly, we found that people's ratings of their ability to effectively increase or decrease emotional expression corresponded with their actual ability to do so in the experiment.[13]

Other research, including further studies from my team, extended this same approach to other kinds of coping and emotion regulation strategies. I've mentioned a few of these studies earlier in the book, when we discussed the flexibility paradox. Across all this work, though, the same basic lesson consistently emerged. The specific strategy was not as important as the extent to which the strategy effectively met the situational challenge.[14] Still, it's important to keep in mind that a good repertoire is not only about coping and emotion regulation strategies. Any behavior, any resource we have at our disposal, is fair game as long as we can use it effectively and as long as it helps us meet the demands of a particular situation.

•

PAUL WAS GOOD at distracting himself. He had no doubts about that. He could become completely absorbed in even the simplest activities.

"I decided I am going to occupy myself. I am going to fill my head. Fill it up. Put anything in there so I could stop thinking about the damn mugging."

And with that, he made himself a drink and sat down to watch a funny movie. It was not exactly a detailed plan, but the fact that he had a plan at all made him feel almost giddy with excitement.

As Paul remembers it, "The movie wasn't great, but it was good enough. It helped that I drank a lot."

Did it work?

"Yeah, actually, well, for a while. The movie made me laugh. That was good. I actually forgot about it for a bit. But, man, the next day, whew, I felt bad. Still, I don't know. I'm not sure how to put it. I had at least done something. I didn't feel any better, but I was different. It's strange to say, even though I was feeling pretty lousy, I was in control. I made myself feel lousy but I made that choice. And I did change the pictures in my head, at least for a bit. At least I was doing something. I was moving forward, and I was going to keep going. I was feeling adamant, almost angry. I was clenching my fist."

This was Paul's confidence and challenge orientation speaking. And, as the day wore on, he used that determined confidence to keep the motivation going. He did some indoor exercises. Jumping jacks, push-ups, sit-ups, as many as he could manage. He bounced around in his apartment to loud music until he was soaked in sweat.

"Yeah, that helped. Moving. It felt good. I was thinking, 'I am going to do this.'"

He went online and tried to distract himself surfing around a bit. That also helped, for a while, until he came across a news story about crime. That stopped him in his tracks.

"I felt it in my gut. I tensed up, immediately. But only at first. I didn't know much about crime. I thought about it. What happens to people like me? People who've been through this? I had no idea. How do people normally react? Does everyone feel this way? I started wondering."

Another thing Paul was good at was research, and soon he set himself the task of finding answers to his questions. If nothing else, it was another distraction. Unfortunately, as Paul quickly discovered, there wasn't much to find on the Internet about men who'd been assaulted. There is no shortage of content about violent acts committed by men, but almost all of it is about violence against women. This is not because men aren't assaulted. Crime statistics, both domestically and internationally, indicate that men actually experience somewhat higher victimization rates than women for all types of violent crime, with the sole exception of sexual assault. Yet information on how male victims react psychologically to violent crime is surprisingly scarce. There are myriad possible reasons for the lack of information, the most likely being that male-on-male violence is often normalized, or dismissed, or simply not even reported.[15]

But there is some research, and that research suggests a portrait of how men react to violent assault that is strikingly consistent with Paul's experience. The most common reactions among victimized men are self-blame, shame, and feeling weak and emasculated. Victimized men are generally reluctant to acknowledge or disclose the experience, even when their lives are severely impacted. They can find it difficult to leave their homes, and frequently they suffer a kind of paranoia, which is centered around suspicions about other people and a fear of repeated persecution.[16]

Unfortunately, Paul never found his way to these studies. Luckily, though, he did come across several websites with firsthand accounts of male victimization that more or less resonated with his own story.

"I devoured it. I couldn't read fast enough. It was like finding a club, people that knew, went through what I was going through.

"It must not seem like much, but for me, man, it was huge, at the time, to see that my reactions were normal. Turns out [chuckles here], I wasn't so pitiful after all. Seriously, though, I can't tell you what it meant. It was a big deal, I could hardly take it in. I still didn't even believe it, not completely. I downloaded the stories. Once I had them, I read them over and over. I tried to let it sink in. I was convincing myself."

Paul was feeling increasingly optimistic. His confidence was bubbling. The hours he'd spent at his computer were a welcome distraction. They also won him some priceless insights and much-needed relief. But the search had been emotional, and Paul decided he deserved a reward. He tried to lose himself in another movie. This time, though, it didn't work. With so much new information floating around in his head, he found he couldn't ignore the fact that he was still sitting in his apartment. He still hadn't gone out.

"I took this huge breath, and then I stood up. 'Stuff those feelings.'" Paul laughs. "I don't know if I really said that, but that's what I felt. I was like, 'Dammit, I am going out.'"

He felt nervous as he opened the door to his apartment, but he was determined to master his fears. And with that, he walked into the hallway, down the stairs, and out onto the street.

Feedback Monitoring

From the moment Paul had his epiphany about the safety of his neighborhood to his abrupt but firm resolve to march himself out onto the street, a full twenty-four hours had passed. During that period, he cycled through many of the tools in his repertoire. He distracted himself, multiple times and in different ways; he engaged in problem-focused reflection; he planned his course of action; he got drunk; he reframed and reappraised; he exercised; and he deliberately suppressed his worry and distress. Most of the time these strategies were effective. Sometimes they were not. Paul was able to make progress, though, because he did more than simply apply the tools in his repertoire. Throughout the twenty-four-hour period, he continually monitored the effectiveness of his behavior, and he modified, updated, and changed it when he needed to.

In doing so, Paul was engaging in the third step of the flexibility sequence, feedback monitoring. The first two steps of the sequence, context sensitivity and repertoire, have us focused on meeting a challenge with the most likely tools we have at our disposal. These two steps take us a long way, but they don't take us all the way. When we engage in the feedback monitoring step, we complete the cycle. Here the question again changes. We are no longer focused on what we need to do or what we are able to do, but on whether whatever we have done is working. In other words, we ask ourselves, "Have I met the challenge?" "Is it working?" "Do I need to adjust my response?" and "Should I try another strategy?" And if a person does try another strategy and is still not getting anywhere, odds are the context has changed, in which case it is necessary to go back to step one of the sequence and reassess the situational context afresh.

We make these judgments based on whatever cues we have. One of the best sources of feedback is right there with us all the time: our own bodies and mental states. In most cases, and in particular in the aftermath of a potentially traumatic event, one's aim is to feel better, to be less anxious, less fearful or sad. In theory, this kind of judgment should be straightforward. We determine whether we are feeling better simply by checking in with ourselves, by paying attention to our emotional states. Unfortunately, that assessment is not always simple or easy.

Many of the reactions we have to the world around us occur without our realizing it. A perfect, albeit mundane, example is the way our bodies regulate internal temperature. The human body is really good at this. Part of the reason is that each of us has literally millions of temperature-sensitive cells, known as *thermoreceptors*, scattered throughout our bodies. Information from these receptors is integrated in a critical structure at the top of the brain stem known as the hypothalamus. If the hypothalamus determines that we are colder than we should be, it signals physiological responses to go into action that help us warm up, such as shivering or vasoconstriction. If we are running hotter than normal, the hypothalamus signals that we need to be cooled down, resulting in sweating, for example, or vasodilation. These internal biological events occur largely without our conscious awareness, which is of course brilliantly efficient because it allows us to focus on other important concerns, like not getting eaten by predators or falling off a subway platform.

By the same token, however, regulating internal temperature only through biological means is costly from a metabolic standpoint. Simply put, biological processes require caloric energy, and caloric energy is expensive. To help defray that cost, and make the process even more efficient, somewhere along the course of evolution animals developed an additional method of temperature regulation: the conscious feeling of being too warm or too cold. These feelings are not necessary, but they are incredibly useful, because they allow animals, including human animals, to change their body temperature simply and efficiently through deliberate behaviors. If we feel too warm, we can take off a sweater, open a window, or turn on a fan or air conditioner.

This same efficiency probably also drove the evolution of threat and fear. Much like temperate regulation, what happens inside us biologically when we react to threat largely occurs without our conscious awareness. When we first encounter a potential threat, before we even quite realize what's happening, our brains will already have activated a rapid, subcortical threat circuit leading to a cascade of biological actions we commonly describe as the fight-or-flight response. The threat circuit doesn't need the conscious experience of fear to do this. Fear is optional. And, actually, it is not even possible for us to experience fear until a bit later in the response chain, after the threat circuit has been activated and its output can be integrated with information from other higher-order cortical regions, such as the dorsolateral prefrontal cortex and the insula.[17] But fear is useful, if not essential. Much as the feeling of being too warm propels us to take off a sweater, the feeling of being frightened propels us to respond to a threat. It rivets our attention to the source of the fear and focuses our thoughts on whatever we might be able to do to survive.

But herein lies the rub. Any emotion, fear included, is adaptive only insofar as it does its job quickly. When fear is prolonged, it becomes unmoored from its original purpose. It diffuses into a general sense of foreboding, an apprehension about what is yet to come. And eventually, if it persists long enough, it morphs into more dysfunctional states, such as anxiety or PTSD. When this happens, decision-making is seriously impaired, and it becomes increasingly difficult, if not impossible, to sort out when our actions are effective and when they are not.[18]

•

PAUL WAS BESET by traumatic stress, fear, and anxious worry in those first days after his assault. It had distorted his perception of himself and the world around him. But because it was still early, he had not yet progressed to full-blown anxiety or PTSD, and he was still able to find his way to using feedback from his own internal states to guide his decisions about strategy change.

To get a better sense of just how common this ability might be, we designed an experiment in which we showed participants a series of photos on a computer monitor, some benign and some disturbing, and instructed them to decrease any negative emotion they felt using a reframing strategy similar to cognitive reappraisal. For example, we told them they could think about how the situation depicted in the photo was not as bad as it first seemed, or imagine ways that the situation could improve for the better. While they were doing this, we monitored their internal state by tracking physiological responses, such as heart rate and facial muscle patterns that had been shown in previous studies to correlate with negative emotions. Reappraisal can be an effective strategy, but it doesn't work as well when emotions are extreme or intense as it does in less intense contexts, and people prefer it less often. A different strategy, such as distraction, tends to be more effective in reducing intense emotions, at least in the short term. To test the ability to make this kind of switch, we repeated the experiment, but this time told participants that four seconds after each photo appeared, they would hear a tone, and at that time they could either continue to use the reappraisal strategy or switch to distraction. As we expected, participants who showed greater distress on the physiological measures were more likely to make the switch. This meant that they were relying on internal feedback to guide that change. Also as expected, some of the participants were more likely to do this than others—that is, they used internal feedback more effectively—and this ability also correlated with better mental health.[19]

In a later study, we extended the same task by providing an external source of feedback: we informed participants that we would tell them directly when they were doing better or worse at regulating their emotions based on readouts from the physiological monitoring equipment. In actuality, and unbeknownst to the participants, the external feedback we provided was bogus. It was completely random and had nothing to do with their actual performance. This meant that they now had a somewhat more difficult task. They had to determine for themselves whether to use our feedback, which was bogus, or their own internal feedback, which was actually reliable. It turned out that participants used the external feedback some of the time, but overall, they still tended to rely on their own more reliable internal information. And, crucially, participants who relied most heavily on that reliable internal feedback were most successful in ultimately keeping their emotional reactions in check.[20]

Although the external feedback we provided in the experiment was bogus, there are genuinely useful sources of external feedback that can help us correct our strategy use. Probably the most meaningful source comes from our perceptions of other people. When we try to learn new behaviors, including basic skills in self-regulation, we learn more effectively when we incorporate social feedback. Individuals who are unable to benefit from such feedback have a notoriously difficult time behaving appropriately in social situations. Autistic individuals, for example, who are known to have difficulty perceiving social feedback, are often unable to change their behavior from one situation to the next. Neuropsychological patients with damage to the orbitofrontal cortex have similar deficits in utilizing social feedback and also have difficulty matching their behavior appropriately to the situational context. From the other extreme, depressed people tend to overreact to social feedback, which in turn leads them to withdraw socially.[21]

•

PAUL WAS NERVOUS about being outside, but he was also determined. It felt good to be there. He walked around his neighborhood for a while and then found his way to an empty bench and sat down. Nothing happened. It almost felt normal. He sat for a while longer, and then he decided to walk to a nearby bodega and pick up some food for later.

"The same guy is always behind the counter. He knows me. I go in there fairly regularly. I could tell he was looking at me when I walked in. Then I remembered about my face, the stitches and all. He said something, I don't remember what, something simple, like, 'What happened to you?' This threw me. All of a sudden, I was super anxious. I said, not sure exactly, I mumbled something about being a klutz and falling. Whatever I said, he seemed okay with it. He kind of laughed, and I kind of laughed, and it was okay. I was feeling pretty shaky. But I got through it."

Leaving the store, satisfied with his accomplishment, Paul turned to walk back home. Then he spotted a group of young men just ahead, gathered near the next corner. They looked a lot like the men who had mugged him, or at least he imagined they did.

"'Oh, shit.' I thought, 'Here we go.' They were just kind of hanging out, but I was sure, I thought, for sure they were watching me."

Paul felt surges of panic.

"I didn't know what to do. I hesitated, just for a second. I couldn't just stop. That would have looked weird. I told myself, 'Just keep going. Go. Walk.'"

Paul was doing his best to conceal his anxiety, but, just as he approached the men, an elderly woman ambled out of a store, directly into his path. He sidestepped her but found himself uncomfortably close to one of the men. To Paul's surprise, the whole group politely backed away so he could pass, and then resumed their conversation as if nothing had happened. Paul chanced a glance over his shoulder. They didn't seem to be paying him much notice.

"Such a relief. I was just relieved, and proud I think, too. It was a small thing. It felt like, 'Okay, I am back out there. This is my neighborhood again.'"

Paul decided to stay out longer. He walked around and eventually made his way back to the same bench and sat down again.

As he basked in the change, it occurred to him that it had been four days since the attack and he had still not contacted his friends to let them know what was going on. And he had not yet called his girlfriend, Carrie.

"Yeah, that was going to be the hard one. She would be kind of pissed. I was sure. She thought I was blowing her off. How could she not? I hadn't told her anything."

Paul took on the easiest challenge first. He contacted his boss and explained about the mugging. He did this by email. It felt safest that way. Then he did the same with some of his friends, including Mark and Laura. He was still sending emails when his phone rang. It was his boss. Paul hesitated, then answered. He was surprised at how obviously concerned and supportive his boss was and at how easy the conversation went. Soon other friends began emailing and calling.

"It happened kind of fast. Before I could even track it. It was a flood. I was talking to people and emailing, for at least an hour. I can't tell you. It felt so good. Everybody was so concerned, and I felt like I was being liberated from this stuff. It's hard to remember exactly. My emotions, they were all over the place. But I think that's when I first stopped feeling like this was my fault, like there was something wrong with *me*. Nobody seemed to think it was my fault. Everyone was being so nice, concerned. And I was thinking, 'Yeah, it's not my fault. Why did I ever think that in the first place?'"

Eventually, Paul was reassured enough to take on the big task. He called Carrie.

"She was upset, just like I expected. Angry at first, that I hadn't called her. But she was good. She is good. She's a kind person. She was crying. I could feel her love through the phone. That was the best thing, really, to feel that."

After he finished talking on the phone and emailing people, Paul sat quietly for a little bit.

"I let out this huge sigh, and just relaxed. I thought to myself, 'Hey, I've been sitting here for a while. Everything is basically okay.' I kind of forgot to be worried. Yeah, I actually felt safe."

Remembering and Reinventing

Paul had transformed the stress that had been plaguing him. He reinvented his memory of the assault. He remade it into something he could live with.

We tend to think of memories as stable facts, unchangeable snapshots that form permanent records of our experiences. In fact, memories are modifiable. When we first create a memory, the various pieces of the experience, the sights, sounds, and thoughts that compose it, are consolidated into a neural pathway in the brain. When we recall that memory, these same neural elements are reactivated. Only the process is not quite as basic as simply pulling a memory from storage. Our brains actively re-create a memory. It is a biological process, one that is influenced by a host of factors, including how strong or accessible the various elements might be, the conditions under which the memory was triggered, and what we might have been thinking or doing at the time of recall. These factors in turn influence not only what we remember but how the memory might change as it is reconsolidated back into an enduring neural pathway.[22]

Paul retained a pretty clear memory of the basic details of his assault. But his flexibility in using different strategies to come to grips with the event helped him to situate himself in a more nuanced narrative. He no longer viewed himself as a pitiful coward who had brought the attack on through his own stupidity. He revised and updated that memory and now saw himself as an innocent person who had experienced a bad event, one to which he had responded in a way that was natural and only to be expected. He realized that most people in the same situation would have responded the same way.

We saw evidence of a similar kind of memory evolution in our 9/11 research. Survivors who had been in or near the towers during the attacks had vivid memories of their experiences. Those who ultimately suffered a trajectory of chronic PTSD symptoms continued to recall roughly the same memories over time. But those who were resilient or showed a recovery trajectory later recalled fewer of the threatening details and over time began to remember the day as more benign than they had originally thought.[23]

The modification of a potential trauma memory has also been demonstrated experimentally. In one study, for example, researchers asked participants to watch a gruesome film. Then, a day later, they reminded them of the film and asked them to recall it as vividly as possible. Afterward, they instructed some of the participants to imagine themselves feeling safe with an important attachment figure: "Someone in your life who is very supportive to you. The person who you would turn to when you need help. Someone who is very close to you and has been there for you when you need them." By imagining themselves with this safe attachment figure, these participants reconsolidated a more benign memory of the trauma film. Over the course of the following week, they recalled less vivid and less distressing memories compared to a control group that did not receive the attachment figure instruction.[24]

•

PAUL'S VICTORY OVER traumatic stress was lasting. But his difficulties were not over quite yet. Once he allowed people back into his life, the changes came fast. Carrie came over later that same day, and although they had a nice evening together, there were a few ups and downs. Fortunately, Paul's boss had told him not to worry about rushing back to work, so he took a few more days to stay at home. As Paul put it, "I practiced going out."

Once he did return to work, and his routine stabilized, Paul discovered that his updated memory of the assault was only a partial fix. It was a long time before he felt comfortable walking alone at night. He often found himself anxiously looking over his shoulder. It was a long time, too, before reminders of the assault completely stopped evoking painful memories and that very unwelcome feeling of shame. Paul did his best to fight off those reactions. Over time, they lessened, although they never quite vanished.

Throughout this period, Paul most likely cycled through the flexibility sequence innumerable times. Was he aware of doing so? It's hard to know. Although his recollections of the first few poignant days after the attack were vivid and detailed, once he resumed his usual life he was just as busy as he had been before the attack, if not busier. His memory from that period was vague, at best.

Which leaves us with some intriguing questions. Was Paul aware of his own flexibility? If he had known more about flexibility at the time, would it have helped him to recast his assault experience more completely, shortened his struggle, or at least made the whole process less onerous? Would it help anyone in that kind of situation to know more?

As long as I've been studying flexibility, I've assumed that these skills would be valuable for just about anyone to learn. Teaching people how they might become more *resilient* has always seemed to me to be out of reach. Resilience is complicated and, as we've seen, hard to predict with any accuracy. We can put a lot of effort into cultivating whatever resilience-promoting traits appear on whatever list we might come across only to discover that we've barely moved the needle. *Flexibility*, on the other hand, gives us something to work with. Although learning to become more flexible doesn't guarantee that a person will be resilient, it does increase the odds, because it gives a person a way to bring all those resilience-promoting traits and behaviors to bear on their situation as best they can, a method not only for working out which traits and behaviors are likely to work best at a given moment but also for correcting and fine-tuning as we go along.

Our research has shown that most people have the ingredients, or at least are capable of cultivating the ingredients, of a flexibility mindset: optimism, confidence in coping, and a challenge orientation. Our research has also shown that most people have at least a moderate level of skill in each part of the flexibility sequence: context sensitivity, a repertoire of tools, and feedback monitoring. These components—the flexibility mindset and the flexibility sequence—tend to co-occur, that is, people who are capable of one also tend to be capable of the other.[25] But, curiously, it also seems to be the case, at least anecdotally, that most people are not aware, or are only minimally aware, of using them in any kind of systematic way. Admittedly, the mindset and the sequence both have a lot of moving parts. But those components are graspable. Actually, the potential *learnability* of these concepts is one of the main reasons I was drawn to study them in the first place. It was also my driving motive for writing this book.

So, how do we do it? How do we learn to be more flexible? We know that most people are at least moderately flexible already, even if they don't know it. So perhaps it would be best to address an even more basic question: How do we become flexible in the first place?

CHAPTER 8

Becoming Flexible

A fter finishing high school, I traveled around the country for
several years and found short stints of employment in fruit
orchards and on farms. One of the farms kept goats. It was my task
to milk them. I knew almost nothing about goats, except that they
had a reputation for being ornery and strong willed. It seemed well
earned, at least for the goats I was trying to milk. Most of the time
I felt I was wrestling more than milking, but eventually I got the
job done.

One morning, as I entered the barn, I witnessed one of the goats
giving birth. Moments later, to my amazement, as the nanny goat
was licking the remnants of amniotic fluid off her newborn, it bayed
loudly, jerked itself up, and walked away. Many mammals are capable of this marvelous feat, I later learned. These creatures are known
as *precocial*, meaning they are more or less born ready to engage with
the world. Humans, by contrast, are *altricial*. The word is derived
from the Latin root *alere*, which means to nurse, support, or suckle.
Newly born humans are almost completely helpless and need to be
cared for over an extended period of infancy before they can even

begin to manage on their own. In fact, everything about human development is extended. We spend almost twice as long in childhood and adolescence as our closest primate relatives do and it takes about twenty-five years—a quarter of a century!—for our brains to fully develop.

There are reasons for the slow course of human maturity. One of the most compelling explanations comes from an unprecedented study of brain data on over seven hundred animal species linking the time required to reach maturity to the number of neurons in the cerebral cortex. According to the study's author, Suzana Herculano-Houzel, "It makes sense that the more neurons you have in the cortex, the longer it should take a species to reach that point where it's not only physiologically mature, but also mentally capable of being independent." The delay, she added, "gives those species with more cortical neurons more time to learn from experience, as they interact with the environment."

The number of cortical neurons also predicts how long a species typically lives. In the case of humans, this, too, makes perfect sense, because, as Herculano-Houzel put it, the cortex "is capable of making our behavior complex and flexible" in a way that "extends well beyond cognition and doing mental math and logical reasoning." Our cortex provides us with a capacity for "adaptability, as it adjusts and learns how to react to stresses and predict them," and "helps keep our internal physiological reactions on track with what you're doing, with how you feel, and with what you expect to happen next."[1]

•

As NEWBORNS, WE begin this elaborative development process with only the most rudimentary ability to self-regulate. We can convey basic social signals, at first mainly crying and smiling, but that's about it. Initially, these signals are more or less undifferentiated. They occur largely in response to internal biological events, such as hunger or gas pain, and have little relation to the outside world. But even in early infancy, as the brain develops further, babies become increasingly responsive to their surrounding environment and their signals become more varied. Within a month or two of birth, the capacity for intentional "social smiling" begins to appear. Caregivers are highly responsive to these expressions and their reactions further shape the infant's expressive behavior. But like all social communication, the influence goes both ways. As neonate researcher Emese Nagy put it, "babies quickly gain a remarkable ability to regulate the behavior of their parents."[2]

From here, the capacity to read and respond to contextual cues—context sensitivity—develops steadily, progressing throughout childhood.[3] With further brain development, reciprocity with the external world expands. The capacity for executive control begins to appear and with it the capacity for planning and monitoring behavior. Children gradually learn the rules and contingencies that inform their actions and, with time, figure out how those rules and contingencies vary across situations. If all goes well, the foundations for context sensitivity are set in place, and by school age, children are able to modify the strategies they use in response to constraints imposed by different situations.

If all does not go well, and the development of context sensitivity is delayed, behavioral problems usually become apparent, even at an early age. In one study, for example, researchers examined fear-related facial expressions and crying in two-year-olds across different types of situations. Most of the children modified their behaviors to at least some degree for different situations, so that their responses depended on how threatening a situation was. There was, however, a small group of "dysregulated" children who showed excessive fear even in the least threatening situations, and these context-insensitive reactions predicted more enduring physiological stress. Another study, this time looking at preschoolers (four- and five-year-olds), linked context insensitivity in emotional behavior with important social costs. Children who displayed greater positive emotions, such as happiness, were generally well accepted by peers, but children who displayed happiness in contextually inappropriate situations, such as in disagreements with other children, were less accepted by peers and also rated by teachers as less socially skilled. The results went in the opposite direction, as would be expected, for anger, a disruptive emotion. Children who displayed greater overall anger were generally less well liked by peers, while children who displayed anger in the more contextually appropriate context of disagreements with other children were not disliked by peers.[4]

A similar trajectory has been observed for the development of a basic coping and emotion regulation repertoire. Infants learn to regulate their distress initially through rudimentary distraction, such as by turning their heads away from unpleasant things or focusing on more desired objects or images. Infants also learn how to use specific behaviors—crying, redirection of the face, eye contact—to elicit helpful responses from caregivers. As toddlers develop increasingly more sophisticated motor control, they also begin to learn how to change stressful situations directly through their own instrumental actions. By preschool, children are learning new ways to distract themselves by manipulating the world around them, such as by keeping busy or playing games. Through the school years, the strategy repertoire expands further. With adolescence, distraction techniques become more sophisticated and include internally generated forms of diversionary thinking. These developmental periods also coincide with the expansion of potential sources of support. In addition to immediate caregivers, teachers and peers begin to play greater roles in the child's life. As their cognitive capacities expand further, children learn to choose between possible sources of support based on contextual cues, such as the degree to which a situation is controllable, or whether or not the adults who are present have clear authority. Cognitive coping skills surge with the onset of adolescence, when it becomes easier to cope more directly through internal problem solving and to use forms of cognitive restructuring, such as reappraisal.[5]

There are clear development markers as well for the third component of the flexibility sequence, feedback monitoring. The foundational skills needed for problem solving and reflective learning first appear in early childhood. By preschool, children can usually modify their problem-solving strategies as needed and will try out new strategies when the old ones are not ideal. This ability of preschoolers to discover alternative problem-solving solutions coincides with a capacity to generate new strategies for regulating emotions. By school age, children show evidence of meta-cognition—an awareness of their own thought processes. By adolescence, meta-cognition is well established and with it the capacity to switch strategies through deliberate cognitive restructuring and corrective reflection.[6]

It takes us a couple of decades to work all this out and to bring these diverse strands in line. It's a long march. Ideally, if all goes well, we progress, as developmental theorists Ellen Skinner and Melanie Zimmer-Gembeck described it, "from diffuse to differentiated, from uncoordinated to integrated, from egocentric to cooperative, and from reactivity to proactive, autonomous regulation." When we reach that end point, as adults, we typically possess the tools to make "an appraisal of the significance of the environmental circumstance, . . . the selection of some action to regulate the heightened emotion and perhaps alter the environment, and some kind of feedback regarding the success of the regulation attempt."[7] In short, the components of flexibility.

The Other Side

The last thing Jed remembered on the night of the accident was saying to his girlfriend, Megan, "I'll see you on the other side." He never imagined just how far away that other side was going to be. The repeated surgeries, the physical adjustments, the years of uncertainty. It was as inconceivable as it was relentless. But Jed never gave up. He got through it and, by all accounts, was doing remarkably well.

We saw brief signs, earlier, that Jed was able to evoke a flexibility mindset even in the turmoil of the hospital on the night of his injury. Having known him now for a number of years, I can say with certainty that he does indeed have a solid flexibility mindset. He is generally optimistic about difficulties. He has a kind of humble confidence in his ability to cope, and he readily focuses on the challenges his life presents him with. It would be inaccurate to say he never had doubts. But he "always knew," he told me, that things "would eventually return to normal."

With a flexibility mindset as part of his nature, Jed was primed to engage the flexibility sequence. He paid attention to the cues. He always had at least some idea of what he needed to do, and he kept himself focused on the tasks at hand. He also had a pretty good idea of what he was good at, the kinds of tools he had in his repertoire. Jed is a highly social being. He's charming and warm in social interactions, but he readily allows himself to take succor in what other people can give him. He uses distraction. He reframes his difficulties, and he focuses on the positive. He jokes around and has a great sense of humor. And he is able to vary his approach. When something isn't working, he changes course.

At one point, a bit down the road of his recovery but before he left the hospital, Jed was moved to an inpatient rehab unit. He shared a room with another amputee, who, as it happened, had lost the opposite leg that Jed had. The irony was palpable. Jed thought so too. He showed me a delightful photo of himself and his roommate, both smiling as they stood side by side, in perfect symmetry, each missing the opposite leg. One day, Jed needed new shoes and realized, he told me with a smile, that he could buy one pair and split them with his roommate. It was dark humor, to be sure, but it also brought some welcome emotional relief.

What got Jed through the entire ordeal, more than anything else, was the support he received from family and friends—in particular, his mother, his sister, and Megan.

"The surgeries were painful and traumatic," he said. "I didn't know if my guts were ever going to work right again. And along the way I thought about Megan and, you know, how her life had been irrevocably altered. It was not what she signed up for."

Jed and Megan had been together for a couple of years when the accident happened. Their relationship was solid, and Jed had been thinking about proposing sometime in the near future. The accident changed everything. From that moment forward, all bets were off. Jed's life had been funneled into one overriding goal: survival. Megan could have moved on, and nobody would have faulted her. But she didn't. She stayed with Jed, and along with his mother and sister formed the core of his support team.

"Their support really carried me. My mom, my sister, and Megan. They were there all the time. In the hospital, when I came out of the coma, they kind of like set up vigil around the clock.

"If I were to catapult myself back to that time, right after coming to, it was like, your whole being was tenuous, there was like this thin veil of awareness. You know, because of what I'd been through, and the medications, it was like I was almost not alive. Barely there. Then Megan would be there. She would come into my consciousness. Almost like light, like soothing consciousness. And my sister and mom, their presence. Their support literally felt physiological, literally like a bridge back to the world."

Jed was still recovering from the prolonged intubation and at this point couldn't yet speak. He used a notepad to communicate, and he still has that notebook. One day he showed me a page in which he had scrawled a note to Megan, his mother, and his sister. It said, "You guys are a great team. I would pick you for any big life events."

That team never faltered. Jed recovered, and two years later, he and Megan were married.

But at that time, he was still not fully out of the woods.

"There were periods off and on where the effects were diminished, but I would say it wasn't until like at least another year that I was actually like okay, you know, when I had passed the major bumps in the road and could focus now on, you know, life as we know it."

For Jed, this meant resuming his studies at City College and eventually completing his master's degree in psychology. But no sooner had he accomplished that goal than he set his sights on an even more ambitious goal, a doctoral degree.

It was sometime after that, about five years after the accident, that I first met Jed. This was when I interviewed him for a slot in our doctoral program. It didn't take me long to decide to accept him into our program, and it didn't take him long to find his bearings. He thrived right from the start, quickly becoming an integral member of my research team. A year later, he and Megan had their first child. Everything was falling into place.

Jed's inspiring success brings us back to the question we asked earlier, about whether or not people are aware of their own flexibility. Although he had become familiar with the tools he had at his disposal, and he was flexible enough to use those tools effectively, Jed barely even knew the concept of flexibility existed. But was that a problem? He had survived an egregious accident and repeated physical and emotional repercussions, and his life was back on track. Does it really matter whether he knew how he did it? It turns out, as we'll see shortly, that it does matter, but with a twist. When we look closely, we see that awareness is not always as clear cut as it might seem.

Conscious or Unconscious

Most people assume that they cope with life's difficulties consciously and deliberately. Many psychologists share this assumption. One influential group of developmental researchers, for example, defined coping as "conscious and volitional efforts to regulate emotion, cognition, behavior, physiology, and the environment in response to stressful events or circumstances."[8]

But is this always the case? Is coping always conscious and deliberate? Part of the reason psychologists might believe so comes from the way we study these processes. We use experiments in which we instruct people to deliberately regulate themselves certain ways. We use survey questionnaires in which we ask people to tell us directly how or when they cope. But if we are always consciously aware of our coping, then we should know a lot about it, and, as we saw earlier, most of us can't actually report on our coping habits with much accuracy.

Flexibility is probably even more elusive. It might seem difficult, if not impossible, to be flexible without knowing it. Yet many people have told me informally that they had no idea they were using anything like the flexibility sequence, or even that such a sequence existed. Does this mean, then, that we can be flexible unconsciously?

•

FOR MANY, THE word "unconscious" still evokes notions of a mysterious reservoir of primitive impulses and urges that we vaguely associate with the writings of Sigmund Freud. We've come a long way since Freud, though. An enormous amount of research in psychology, neuroscience, biology, and psychiatry has helped clarify how our brains process information, both with and without conscious awareness. As we discussed previously, most of what goes on in our brains occurs without our having any conscious knowledge of it at all. But we are conscious beings, and when we think about something consciously, a lot can happen. Most importantly, in terms of flexibility, we can change the way we use information.[9]

Psychologists have known about the basic components of this kind of information change for a long time. In the 1970s, a great deal of research focused on what eventually came to be called *automatic and controlled processes*. An automatic process usually happens quickly and requires no attention or conscious control on our part, and, once activated, it can be difficult to interrupt or ignore. For example, a red stop light can trigger an automatic braking response from a driver. Even if the driver realizes too late that the light is changing, and decides to run the red light, she may still automatically experience a twitch in the leg that would normally be used to apply the brakes. By contrast, a controlled process is always instigated by deliberate conscious intention. Controlled responses are slower, more effortful, and more limited than automatic ones, because of the amount of conscious attention they require. It is also easier to interrupt a controlled process, and controlled processes can be interrupted by automatic processes.[10]

It's reasonable to think of automatic processes as unconscious, at least when they are initiated. But in this case the word has a somewhat different meaning from the classic Freudian unconscious. In the Freudian unconscious, thoughts and behaviors are banished to the nether regions of our minds and plague us in disguised form until we make them conscious. But automatic processes, as an abundant body of research has shown, typically follow the opposite route. They begin as deliberate, conscious thoughts and behaviors, and, with time and repetition, eventually become automated and nonconscious.

To return to the driving example: We are not born knowing how to drive a car. It's actually a rather unnatural, complex activity. We have to first learn several unique behaviors, and then we have to get used to performing them simultaneously. We need to integrate various movements of our hands and feet, for example, with judgments about visual distances and the presence or absence of other cars or other possible obstacles. Initially, driving seems impossible. I can still vividly remember practicing on a simulator in my high school driver education class and repeatedly failing to brake for pedestrians or objects that appeared on the screen. I was horrified by my failures—my car simulator plowed right through everything in sight—but, like most would-be drivers, eventually I learned.

With practice, for most people driving a car becomes second nature. We can hold conversations or listen to the radio while still monitoring the car's speed, tracking other cars, and braking for objects in the road. In short, much of the process becomes automated, so automated that we can practically do it in our sleep. And sometimes, research has shown, we actually do sleep, at least for brief moments, while driving.[11] Thankfully, it would be impossible to drive unconsciously for very long. As overlearned as it might be, like all complex behavior sequences, driving a car still requires conscious monitoring. We need to periodically and consciously track our speed, for example. We need to take deliberate actions at specific decision points, such as when to make a turn, or whether to pass another vehicle. And we always need to be aware of unexpected obstacles and changes in the roadway and be ready to respond.

It's easy to imagine that similar contingencies would apply to the flexibility sequence. As we've already seen, we aren't born with the skills that make up the sequence. We have to learn each individual component, consciously, deliberately, and often painstakingly. For most children, it's a demanding process. Decoding situational cues, reeling in impulses and managing emotions, correcting and adjusting: these are all genuine skills that initially require guided instruction from parents or other adults along with a great deal of trial-and-error practice. As we grow older, and our brains develop, these skills become easier. With time, they even become partially automated. Yet, as we've seen, each of the individual components only gets us so far. Even the best coping strategies or the most razor-sharp assessments of contextual cues are only so effective. Flexibility involves coordinating the different skills, tracking them, and adjusting and changing them as we go along, and these processes require at least some conscious monitoring. Without it, our capacity to adapt ourselves quickly gets off track.

•

WE LIVE OUR lives in a constantly evolving context. Most of the situations we encounter during our normal, daily routines, such as sitting down to eat, or saying hello to a neighbor, or checking email, are fairly mundane and predictable. The cues about what might be happening in these situations, and how we should respond, are usually so obvious that we scarcely even notice them. Or at least we don't realize we notice them. Not every situation is so readily discernible, of course. When we find ourselves in a new or unusual situation, we typically need to focus our thought processes and to consciously pay attention to whatever cues might be available to guide our behavior. Even then, we can easily miss important information, or misunderstand the cues we do perceive.

One of the primary reasons we might fail to adequately decode a situational context, even when we are paying attention, is that we can only do so much consciously at any given time. Conscious awareness is limited. There is an enormous body of research attesting to this fact. And you can easily demonstrate it for yourself. Take a moment and try to count backward by threes from the number 1,754. Make sure to keep your eyes open while you do. You don't need to go all the way to zero. Just try it for a few seconds. It's difficult, but by no means impossible. Now, if you are willing, try counting backward again, and this time close your eyes. It's easier. That's because there is less you can consciously attend to—there is no visual input—and you have more conscious attentional resources available for the task of counting backward.

Okay, now let's switch to a different task. Try picking out all the verbs on the page you are reading. This is moderately difficult, depending on your facility with grammar, but it's also doable. Now, try picking out the verbs on the page while at the same time counting backward. That is all but impossible. The reason is that both of these tasks—identifying verbs and counting backward—require conscious resources, and we simply don't have enough of those resources to do both tasks at the same time.

The story is similar when we try to consciously scan and decode the contextual cues around us. If we are doing absolutely nothing else, the process is not difficult. But if we are consciously busy with other activities—such as trying to solve a problem, anticipating a future event, worrying, or talking with someone—then we have fewer available conscious resources, and it becomes much more likely that we'll miss important contextual cues.

The limited scope of what we can do consciously is actually the most plausible argument for why it would be advantageous, on some level, to automate some aspects of the flexibility sequence, such as decoding contextual cues. Automated processes are fast and easy, and they help us efficiently make decisions about the world around us. And in fact, children show evidence of automatic context perception even at an early age, and then their automatic context perception improves throughout the course of development.[12]

But there is a potentially serious drawback to relying too much on automatic processing: it's not always accurate. Even when we are consciously paying attention to the contextual cues, we still tend to process some cues automatically or nonconsciously, and, as we saw earlier with heuristic shortcuts, that can result in potentially serious misinterpretations. These kinds of errors are especially likely when we are pressed to make rapid decisions, which is often the case when we are in dangerous or stressful situations.

A classic example of automatic cue perception interfering with a conscious decision comes from a classic experiment known as the Stroop Color and Word Test. The task is deceptively simple. Research participants are shown a series of words, one at a time, with each word appearing in a different color. For example, the word "house" in red letters, followed by the word "dog" in blue letters. The task is simply to identify the color of the letters for each word as quickly and accurately as possible. Pretty easy. That is, as long as the words are common, uninteresting words, such as house or dog, and easily ignored. But what if the words are color names? In this case, the meaning of the words automatically cues additional relevant information. That's because reading is a highly practiced skill that is, for most literate people, automatic. If a word spells a color name that is the same as the color of the letters (the word "blue" in blue letters), then it will automatically speed up how fast we can name the color. But, crucially, if the word spells a competing color (the word "blue" in red letters), then we have conflicting information and will be measurably slower to name the color of the letters. That's because we need extra time and must make more of an effort to resolve the discrepancy. Usually, this task takes at least some conscious attention.

A disturbing real-world example of this same kind of unconsciously cued interference comes from research on automatic racial stereotypes. In a classic study, research participants were repeatedly shown two pictures, one after the other, on a computer monitor. They were instructed to always ignore the first picture, which was always a face, and to pay attention only to the second picture. The task was to determine, as quickly and accurately as possible, whether the second picture depicted a gun or a tool. The experiment was designed to study automatic racial stereotypes. The participants were always white, the first picture was always a photo of either a white male or a black male face, and it was always flashed very briefly, only a fifth of a second, which is barely enough time to consciously notice the color of the face, but plenty of time for our brains to process it automatically. The findings were striking. When the white participants were flashed the black male face, they were subsequently faster to correctly identify photos of guns, but they were also, crucially, more likely to misidentify some of the tool photos as guns. This is a powerful effect. Only a brief flash of an unknown black male face was enough to automatically cue a racial stereotype associating black males with guns, and that stereotype was strong enough to tilt the white participants' perceptions of context in the direction of danger. A racial bias was also observed for white male faces, only in this case the bias went in the opposite direction. A brief flash of a white male face automatically cued contextual perceptions of safety.[13]

There is also evidence for automatic processing in relation to the repertoire component of the flexibility sequence, but the same dangers of automatic mistakes as well. In one study, a group of participants were primed unconsciously to use cognitive reappraisal, while another group was told explicitly to use that strategy. The group that was primed for automatic reappraisal did just as well in coping with a highly stressful task—their physiological reactivity during the task was just as low—as the group that was explicitly instructed to reappraise.[14]

But although these results show clearly that, at least in some circumstances, we are capable of engaging in a specific regulation strategy automatically, what is not clear is how often we would actually be able to take advantage of that process. More importantly, from the perspective of flexibility, automatic strategies would have obvious limitations. As we've seen repeatedly, no strategy, including reappraisal, is always adaptive. In situations where we have some control over the stressor, reappraising away our emotional reactions has been found to be somewhat ineffective and even potentially harmful, because it keeps us from effectively engaging in problem-solving strategies. Most other strategies come with similar drawbacks. For example, automatically suppressing a threatening emotion might make us feel better, but, as we saw earlier, in some situations the conscious awareness of threat is vital for survival.

This is why the third step of the flexibility sequence, feedback monitoring, is so important. When a strategy is not working, feedback, either from our bodies or from the world around us, tells us that we need to either modify the strategy or try something else. But if the strategy had been activated automatically, the monitoring and adjusting process might not actually come online. Indeed, one series of studies showed that even when an automatically activated strategy helped reduce participants' distress, they had no awareness of the change.[15] And if a strategy is helping us and we don't know it, we might inadvertently switch to another, less effective strategy. The lack of awareness could be especially problematic when an automatic strategy is not appropriate for a specific situation. If we have no awareness of whether something is helping us, we can't correct it or even deliberately keep doing it. There is some evidence to suggest that, under the right circumstances, we might be able to automate the strategy correction process.[16] But regardless of whether that can occur, the evidence we have clearly indicates that feedback correction is largely a conscious decision. In other words, we need to be paying attention. And at no time is this more the case than when we are hit with unexpected challenges. When we are caught off guard by a major stressor, we definitely need to be paying attention.

Nightmare Redux

Which brings us back, once again, to Jed. Sadly, as much as he had already been through, Jed had another unexpected trial looming on his horizon. Even worse, this new challenge was in many ways more distressing and demanding than his previous troubles. It all began with a lingering problem that at first seemed manageable.

When a limb is amputated, naturally all sensory input from that limb is lost. Yet amputees often continue to experience the missing limb as if it were still there. Unfortunately, that experience can involve severe pain. It was once assumed that phantom limb pain was a psychological phenomenon, a kind of hallucination that could be treated with psychological interventions. But phantom limb pain is actually physiological. When a limb is amputated, the nerve fibers that once carried sensory information from the limb to the spinal cord, and ultimately to the brain, are severed. But although those nerves are damaged, the pathways from what remains of the nerves to the brain still exist. This means that the brain can interpret any stimulation of the remaining nerve as coming from the amputated limb. And because the nerves are damaged, and not functioning as they should, they are often hyperexcitable. Sometimes they form small tumors, called *neuromas*, at the site of the damage. Neuromas exacerbate the sensation of pain.[17]

Jed began experiencing the phantom limb soon after the accident, when he was still in the hospital.

"When I first woke up in the hospital, I felt like my entire leg was there," he said. "It was odd, I felt like my leg was bent at the knee, with my foot going through the hospital bed, but it, my foot, was turned around backward. It wasn't like I imagined it. I knew my leg was gone, but the signals, my brain, it felt super weird, there was this phantom limb. Like if you pay attention to a part of your body, you can feel it, your brain knows it's there. That's what it was like. It wasn't like flesh and bone. More like a hologram. I could sense my whole leg, except the foot was reversed."

As his condition improved, the sensation of the missing leg, the phantom limb, didn't appear to be going away. It looked like Jed had no choice, at least for the moment. He was going to have to get used to it. And gradually he did.

"The only part that tripped me up was getting out of bed, or moving in bed, rolling over, because a quarter of my body weight was gone. I knew it was gone, but my brain was still thinking it was there, so I needed to learn to adjust to that.

"It's very strange. The feeling is nervy. That's the best way to describe it. Like, when I see a cockroach, my whole hip lights up, like a Christmas tree. Like white light. You know, it's just like nerves."

With time, phantom limb pain does tend to improve. The way it does this can be rather bizarre. Jed's experience, which is not uncommon among amputees, was that the phantom limb was gradually shortening. It was as if his missing foot was moving up his missing leg, a phenomenon known as *telescoping*.

"I could always feel all five toes, those first years. But my foot slowly traveled up, so for a while I basically had the sensation that I had like a femur and then my leg stopped at the knee but I still had five toes there. It's a generally good sign when you have telescoping because I think it's a sign of cortical rewiring, you know, somatosensory remapping. But now all I have left, if I pay attention to it, are two phantom toes here [points to end of hip] and a little bit more. I can feel them. I can almost flex them."

Unfortunately, despite the gradual diminution, Jed continued to experience acute pain. And it was becoming a serious problem.

"It had been getting better over time, but still there were flare-ups, intermittent flare-ups, where I would be sleepless for a few nights in a row because of the pain. It always bothered me most at night, as I am falling asleep. Usually, even when it was acute, I could distract myself, you know with headphones or a game, but when I was falling asleep, there were no distractions, and I became more aware of my body. But it also felt physiological. You know, when I lay down, I could feel it ramping up."

Phantom limb pain is still poorly understood. Trying to find a way to ease the problem, Jed consulted with various pain experts. They tried different approaches, including cauterizing the nerve endings, injecting nerve blocking agents (to anesthetize the area of the injury), freezing an area to kill a nerve, and, in several epidural trials, inserting an electrode in the dura layer around the spine near the site to overwhelm the circuitry. Every option was risky, because the injury was located near sensitive areas of the spine. And none of these interventions seemed to be helping with the pain.

Then, in the spring of 2016, everything fell apart.

Jed had begun working with another specialist who had proposed using a brand-new procedure, just approved by the US Food and Drug Administration (FDA). For a normal epidural, an electrode is placed near the outer membrane—the dura layer—of the spine to interrupt nerve transmission and quiet the pain. This procedure is often ineffective because it is not very specific in reference to the damaged area. The new procedure aimed to be more precise by inserting an electrode close to the site of the relevant nerves. This was even riskier than a normal epidural, however, because it targeted the dorsal root ganglia, which is an extremely important and vulnerable component of the nerve emerging from the spinal cord. The fact that the procedure was so new also made it risky. At that point, Jed's doctor had only used the procedure on one other patient.

The first attempt with Jed was unsuccessful. The placement was too high up the spine to make any difference, and the pain continued. Several months later, they tried again.

This time, the consequences were disastrous. The needle used to insert the electrode tore a small hole in the dura layer of Jed's spine, resulting in a subdural hematoma. Blood was seeping into Jed's spinal column. This created a clot, then a cyst, and ultimately leakage of cerebrospinal fluid (CSF). Jed began experiencing strange neurological reactions. These were troubling but manageable at first. Then gradually they got worse. Jed struggled throughout this period but somehow got by.

One of the most vivid memories I have of Jed during this time was an evening when he and I and several other members of my research team attended a concert at one of the downtown clubs. Because there was only limited seating, we had to stand. The club was dark. Jed's face was only partially visible in the flashing colors of the stage lights, but I could still see that he was uncomfortable. He didn't yet know what was happening to him, or whether it had anything to do with the new spinal procedure. He tried to tough it out, but eventually had to leave early.

Sometime later, Jed was working alone in my lab when he began to experience, as he put it, "all these crazy symptoms, like heat and cold up and down my body, and all kinds of weird nerve effects going on."

From that point on, the symptoms worsened at an accelerated clip.

"I was at the hospital doing an externship and I had like this episode where I was all of a sudden super crazy dizzy. I couldn't work, and from that time on, I couldn't really be vertical. I had to lie down, like for several months. . . . That began this really, I mean first of all it was terrifying. It was terrifying to all of a sudden be so really, really off. My vision was off. My balance was off. My heart, all these things. The symptoms were just awful. Headaches, brutal headaches, unremitting headaches. Nausea. I felt like I was going to vomit. I mean, I went to the ER and they thought I had had a stroke."

To make matters even more challenging, only days after Jed returned home from a five-day stay in the hospital for evaluation, he and Megan's second child was born. What would have normally been a full-on joyous occasion was tempered by the confusing weight of Jed's mysterious decline in health. Even worse, the doctors had nothing conclusive to tell him. His instructions were only to take caffeine, which would promote vasoconstriction and presumably help close the leak, and to continue lying down as much as possible. That was it.

"At least it made the pain, the dizziness, all of the symptoms, improve. They weren't gone, but they became tolerable, while I was lying down. But anytime I got up, I would have this acute reversal. All the symptoms. Everything was immediately off again. I literally could do nothing else but lie down."

The change came as a crushing blow. After all he had been through, and just when it seemed he might finally be in the clear, Jed again found himself struggling just to survive. How could it not have been profoundly depressing?

"You know, I don't know what to call it. I mean it wasn't really depression, but if you start to pull back from the things that give you joy, give you a sense of competency, what's the word, your own mastery, your daily life, slipping away, and you know, you're going to start. I mean, yeah, sure, my mood was really shitty. My outlook was really bad, because I didn't know. I just didn't know."

This time Jed really didn't know. His world was slipping away. His mood was spiraling, and he had no idea how to stop it. More than ever, he needed answers. That burning question that started it all—Why was I doing okay?—was still burning. He had only partially answered it. But now, with the stakes higher than ever, it seemed that if he didn't find a more satisfying answer soon, that question might just consume him.

PART V

Repeat After Me

CHAPTER 9

Talking to Ourselves

D r. Wendy Lichtenthal sees a lot of distress and confusion. Wendy is an attending psychologist at Memorial Sloan Kettering Cancer Center in New York City, and many of her patients struggle with unexpected, unwanted, and wholly undesirable challenges. She is always on the lookout for new methods that might help them help themselves.

I first met Wendy years ago, back when she was a doctoral student at the University of Pennsylvania. I had given a talk at the university, and Wendy and I had chatted afterward. I was struck, even then, by her passion to bring science to bear on difficult clinical questions. We kept in touch and eventually she moved to the New York area.

A few years back, I published a paper on the flexibility sequence, although at the time I wasn't yet using that phrase. Wendy read it and got in touch, saying that the strategies I was talking about were exactly what her patients needed. Often her patients had a hard time understanding what was happening to them or figuring out what they could do about it. And in the face of that kind of uncertainty, "they want direct guidance," as Wendy put it. "They say things like, 'Tell me how to cope with this. What's the best way?' But there is no 'best way' because the contexts vary so much for each person, even day-to-day." Wendy thought the flexibility sequence offered a model that she could use to teach them how to find their own paths through their challenges.

Sometime later, Wendy contacted me again to say that, with our discussion on her mind, she had decided to try explaining the flexibility sequence directly to one of her patients, a young mother diagnosed with breast cancer. Her patient was struggling to manage both her anxiety and the well-being of her children while at the same time tending to her own health-care needs. She was feeling overwhelmed and searching for a way to deal with the chaos and stress. Wendy explained to her that in situations like hers, "there is no technical playbook," but that a flexibility framework can help. That is, she could assess whatever was happening in a given context, attempt a strategy pulled from her repertoire, and then assess how well it was working, and if it wasn't, "rinse and repeat" until she struck upon "a strategy that does work." Wendy also explained one of the core assumptions about flexibility, suggesting to her patient that "she may notice that because the context is ever-changing, that what worked yesterday may not help her meet her goals today—being flexible in her approaches is what might be most helpful in this uncharted terrain." Her patient's reaction was unambiguously positive, Wendy told me. "She started taking notes and saying how helpful it was, literally, as we spoke."

It's hard to judge from one example, but Wendy has since continued exploring and fine-tuning ways she might apply the sequence with her patients. Recently, she has found that an understanding of the flexibility sequence is particularly helpful with patients who are waiting for crucial test results. This can be an incredibly stressful situation. For most people, it seems as though "there is nothing they can do. No obvious problem to solve. It's just about waiting."

The flexibility sequence breaks it down into more manageable pieces. For starters, thinking about the context, the situational demand, reveals that there is in fact a problem to solve: keeping oneself from becoming overwhelmed. Then, there is the question of how to address that problem. An obvious strategy would be to use distraction to avoid thinking about the test. Wendy agrees, but also cautions that how this might be communicated is important. True to the flexibility concept, she stresses to her patients that distraction—or any other kind of avoidance—isn't the only approach, and isn't always the best approach.

"For me, language does a lot," Wendy said. "If we say 'distract,' there is an underlying communication that feelings are bad. And we never want to do that. We want to promote the capacity to deal with feelings *when* it's important to do so. Instead of using the word 'distraction,' I'll ask, 'What can you engage in? What can engage your attention? What is meaningful and important to you that, you know, that can light you up?' Inevitably, of course, unwanted thoughts are going to intrude. It would be strange if someone didn't think about this at all. The holy grail is that ability to be able to tolerate the feelings when you need to, but also to be able to move your attention when it's not going to help you."

Expressing that anxiety can also be important. Wendy guides her patients to think about different contexts when it might be safer to let themselves more fully express their worries. Not surprisingly, given the prominent role social support plays in these kinds of situations, the contexts that most often come up are those in which a patient is with someone they are close to. But here, Wendy also emphasizes how important it is for the patient to monitor feedback, both their own internal states and the reactions of the people to whom they might be expressing their distress.

"When a person wants to let out how anxious they are, it can easily turn into this repeated loop, 'I'm so anxious, I'm so scared. I'm so anxious, I'm so scared.' Eventually there is a point where that ventilation doesn't yield anything, where they end up ruminating, but also taxing their support network."

This is, again, where a patient will need to look back to his or her repertoire, to come up with other strategies. This is easier said than done, unfortunately, for patients struggling with life-and-death situations. A common response Wendy hears from her patients is that they just don't know what else they can do.

When this happens, she tries to help them explore what might be possible. It's not always a simple process, she's learned, as there are usually a couple of significant stumbling blocks to get past first. One hurdle is simply the belief many patients have that they are not capable of much else.

"I might say, for example, 'Let's talk about the use of meditation.' A common response I'll hear is, 'I can't do that.' So then I'll try to remind them that Buddhist monks have been training their entire lives, and many still can't meditate very well. Nobody can do anything perfectly. But we can try. We can try to build a skill set. It's all about practice and building skills."

Another common hurdle for many patients is that confronting the immediate situation leads to a kind of existential dread. Life-threatening medical events often instigate profound thoughts about human mortality.

"Beyond the obvious evolutionary explanation that we are scared out of our minds when we are waiting for a test result, there is also the bigger existential implication that 'Life is short, and I've just been reminded of that, and what am I doing with my time, and how am I going to live my life?'"

As big as such existential questions are, we don't often ponder them. But in provocative moments, such as when we're waiting for potentially dreaded news from a medical test, we are compelled to do so.

"You have to think about it. You can't ignore it. But it's like staring at the sun. You can't do it for too long, either."

To help her patients get past these hurdles and expand their repertoire, Wendy sometimes reviews existing lists of self-regulation strategies. Such lists are readily available, and the strategies are often prescribed by different therapy approaches. But as we saw a few chapters back, some of the skills and attributes that find their way onto the various lists are not necessarily helpful for extreme or potentially traumatic and stressful events. When I asked Wendy about this limitation, her response was insightful.

"It's hard to think clearly in the midst of a crisis. When I am working with someone formally, when they are not in a crisis moment, then I have a broader span of time to help them figure out how they might best cope," she said. "I can help them work out their options, create their own personal list of the things that seem to work best for them, whether it's listening to music, or going for a walk, or talking with someone, or distracting themselves with a book or movie. Whatever works for them. But when someone is in an acute crisis situation, where you have a kind of physiological surge, thinking about 'What do I do here?' is not easy. With all that is going on, they just can't access it. They're overwhelmed. And if they haven't even thought about it before, it really helps to start with an established list."

·

Wendy and a colleague, Holly Prigerson, a well-known end-of-life care specialist and bereavement researcher, have developed a more formal intervention to teach aspects of flexibility to a group that sorely needed it: surrogate decision-makers in the hospital's intensive care unit (ICU). When an ICU patient is unconscious or unable to communicate with the medical staff, a surrogate family member is usually enlisted to take over that role. The task can be highly stressful. It often includes the daunting responsibility of making end-of-life decisions on the patient's behalf. Not surprisingly, surrogates report experiencing waves of grief and traumatic stress as well as guilt, regret, and intense anxiety about the choices they are tasked with making. To make matters worse, not knowing what else to do, surrogate decision-makers often channel their anxieties into unnecessary battles with the medical staff regarding the patient's treatment, which only exacerbates the problem.

"The medical team can be the most caring medical team in the world," Wendy explained, "but they know where the treatment is going, and usually they know what the outcome is going to be. They don't have the same emotional experience as the family member, so they often make recommendations that the family member doesn't want to hear or simply can't accept, and it becomes a power struggle."

Earlier attempts to intervene with surrogate decision-makers consisted largely of family meetings with a specialist in palliative care. The meetings were intended to be supportive and informative.

"It was all sensible stuff they were talking about," Wendy explained, "like 'Let's plan this out, talk about what you want and what they want. The goals of care.' But this only made surrogates more distressed."

There was never actually any definitive evidence that the family intervention approach was helpful. Then it was tested in a randomized clinical trial, the gold standard for any kind of treatment. Not only did the intervention fail to reduce the surrogates' depression and anxiety, it actually increased their PTSD symptoms.[1]

At one point, frustrated and out of ideas, the medical staff asked Holly Prigerson for assistance.

As Wendy explained it, "Basically, the ICU physicians said, 'Help, we have these family members who are pushing for aggressive care, intensive interventions that are no longer appropriate. They are fighting us, and the dynamics are awful. It's bad for our clinicians and, obviously, it's horrific for them.'"

Together Wendy and Holly pondered what they might do that would be both practical and possible to help these surrogates. Wendy said, "A surrogate in this situation is like a deer in headlights. The physician is talking to them, and they're dissociating; they're so stunned they're not taking in any of the information. It's all emotion, every kind of emotion. But there are absolutely times when they need to be focusing on a practical matter in the ICU, and so they need to be able to shift away from the grief and emotion."

Wendy and Holly reasoned that this was essentially a question of flexibility. And to inculcate at least some aspects of flexibility, they designed a brief intervention consisting of three sessions.[2] The first session was the longest. It began by establishing a kind of context sensitivity. They laid out the situation and the problem in a rough sketch of the emotional tug-of-war that was looming ahead. This session also included a series of short repertoire-expanding modules that taught the surrogates some of the different tools they might use to help themselves manage their complex task. Two additional sessions were then scheduled, each two weeks apart and conducted by phone. These were essentially feedback monitoring sessions that allowed surrogates to check in with the team to let them know how they were doing, rehearse the strategies they'd learned, and update if needed.

Wendy and Holly's intervention was a big step forward. It demonstrated that it was possible to teach some of the basics of the flexibility approach even in a high-stress context. We have to acknowledge, though, that it could not have been easy. When we are overwhelmed by stress, our resources are already depleted, and it's often hard to think clearly. A less taxing approach, and one that would engender a wider learning experience, would be to practice and enhance the capacity for flexibility in the course of normal daily life, when we are not overcome by stress.

Shoring Up

The flexibility mindset is a good place to begin. To refresh your memory, a flexibility mindset comprises three interrelated beliefs—optimism, confidence in coping ability, and a challenge orientation—that coalesce into an overarching conviction that we will be able to do whatever is necessary, adapting ourselves flexibly, to overcome a demanding challenge.

A number of different approaches have demonstrated that it is possible to effectively increase one's optimism. In one study, for example, researchers used a "best-possible-self" technique in which people imagined themselves "in a future in which everything has turned out as good as possible." While doing this, they wrote down the goals, skills, and desires they wanted to have in the future, and then continued imagining themselves this way on their own. Two weeks later, those who engaged in the best-possible-self technique were more optimistic on several different measures compared to a control group of people who did not engage in the technique.[3]

Shoring up confidence in one's coping ability requires more of an experiential approach that focuses on actual successes. One such approach uses affirmative writing exercises to improve confidence levels, in which participants describe times when they coped effectively. More situation-specific approaches have also been effective, such as directly teaching people coping behaviors tailored to the specific problems they face. Groups as disparate as rugby players and chronic asthma patients have reported greater confidence in their ability to cope after practicing these methods. Research has also shown that it is possible to increase confidence in coping even while highly stressful situations are in progress. For example, in one study, university students who had experienced lasting distress after exposure to mass violence became more confident in their coping ability after several days of engaging in writing exercises tailored specifically toward engendering a sense of mastery and coping efficacy.[4]

The enhancement of challenge orientation works largely the same way. When we succeed in a difficult task, for example, the sense of mastery we feel will tend to carry over to influence subsequent task performance. Educators are well aware of the importance of such generative experiences and have developed various methods of orienting both students' and teachers' appraisals in the direction of challenge and mastery.[5] Experimental studies have also shown that simply instructing participants to think of a pending stressor as a challenge can be enough to activate the physiological coping advantages associated with a challenge orientation.[6]

What about the steps of the flexibility sequence? One series of studies demonstrated how people can learn to use new strategies in response to specific contextual cues. This type of learning has been described as "if-then implementation," which means that if the situational cue is present, then one implements the strategy. In one study using this approach, participants were shown a set of pictures, some neutral, some pleasant, and some with disgusting images, such as mutilations and bloody scenes of burn victims. One group of participants simply viewed the photos, while another group mentally repeated a basic goal of not getting disgusted. The members of a crucial third group repeated an if-then-implementation statement to themselves: "I will not get disgusted, and if I see blood, then I will stay calm and relaxed." Only the participants who learned the if-then-implementation strategy were able to reduce their emotional responses to the disgusting photos.[7]

It is also possible to enhance the effectiveness of specific strategies that people already use. In my own research, colleagues and I adapted the expressive flexibility task I described earlier to measure how well people can modulate their feelings. In one study, we extended the task so that it lasted twice as long as before and discovered that participants were getting better at it over time. Only depressed people failed to improve, which makes sense, given other research showing that depression impedes learning. For everyone else, we found that the ability to modulate between strategies was a skill that could be improved with practice.[8]

Practice can also enhance the use of reappraisal. One group of researchers had participants learn different kinds of reappraisal self-statements, such as, "Bad things happen in the world, and I need to put them behind me and move on," and, "There are usually some good aspects in every situation, and it's important to focus on these." Next, they practiced using these statements during and after viewing a series of disturbing films. After some time had passed, they were shown an additional disturbing film as a test. Compared to a control group, whose members simply watched the films, the participants who practiced the reappraisal self-statements felt less distressed and showed less physiological reactivity during the test film.[9] Another study showed that the benefits of a single session of reappraisal practice lasted for at least several weeks.[10]

Although the resources we use to cope with adversity, such as social support, are usually relatively stable, these, too, can, in some cases, be deliberately enhanced. Training and intervention programs have demonstrated that it's possible to enhance supportive resources in the context of specific problems, such as living with chronic disease or attempting to quit smoking.[11] However, simpler methods have also shown promise. One study found, for example, that a relationship-focused gratitude and kindness exercise improved subsequent relationship satisfaction and perceived friendship. In one of these exercises, participants were told to "write and deliver a positive message to someone in your social network thanking or praising them for something you are grateful for"; in another, they were instructed to "do something kind for someone in your social network." Although the researchers did not assess changes in social support, it seems likely that the boost to relationship quality would exert a positive effect on supportive resources.[12]

Self-Talk

An even simpler approach, and one that can potentially enhance the dynamic interaction of both the flexibility mindset and the flexibility sequence, involves a common technique known as *self-talk*. We already saw a variant of this approach in one of the reappraisal studies we discussed (the one that had participants repeat reappraisal self-statements such as "Bad things happen in the world, and I need to put them behind me and move on").

Self-talk has proved to be an effective learning tool across a range of applications, including education, sports, and mental health. It often goes by different names, such as *self-verbalization* or *inner speech*. Regardless of what we call it, the key idea is that self-talk simplifies complex concepts down to just a few words. We often do this spontaneously and automatically, without even realizing it, and not infrequently with a heavy dose of emotion. Consider, for example, when someone suddenly realizes the correct answer to a confusing test question. Or perhaps she makes a difficult basketball shot, or discovers that her dinner guests loved a meal that she cooked. The self-talk in these cases might be something along the lines of "I've been working hard on this. I've been worried. I thought it might be more than I can handle. But I actually managed to pull it off." Except that it's actually much briefer: it pops into our consciousness in a simplified version of this entire thought process, something like a single, emphatic word, "Yes!" But there is also a darker side to spontaneous self-talk. It can be negative as well as positive. To use the same example, we might fail the test question, miss the basketball shot, or watch in anguish as our dinner guests push aside the meal. In these cases, we might tell ourselves something like, "Dummy," or "I should have known."

Self-talk is most effective as a learning tool when it is used intentionally. This is sometimes referred to as *goal-directed self-talk.* There is a big difference between spontaneous and goal-directed self-talk. Spontaneous self-talk is best understood as an expression of an underlying psychological process that has automatically broken into conscious awareness. Goal-directed self-talk, in contrast, is a controlled form of inner speech that we deliberately engage in to facilitate a psychological process or skill. And it has proved effective for skills that are highly relevant to the components of flexibility we've been discussing, such as regulating appraisals, strengthening confidence, facilitating strategic decision-making, increasing effort, controlling emotion, and modifying or adjusting strategy use.[13]

When we tailor goal-directed self-talk specifically to the flexibility mindset, it takes the form of an affirmative monologue in which we repeat to ourselves statements that remind us about, and reinforce, each of the three beliefs that make up the mindset. To activate the motivating effects of optimism, for example, we might say to ourselves, "The future will be okay." To foster confidence in our coping ability, we might tell ourselves, "I have the skills to get the job done." And to orient ourselves to the challenge at hand, we might say, "I will do what is necessary."

These simple statements by themselves do not make us optimistic, or confident, or oriented to the challenge. What they do is remind us that we can use these beliefs to help cultivate optimism, confidence, and orientation to a challenge. And if you are not sure whether or not you possess these beliefs, you can practice this kind of self-talk informally to cultivate the mindset. You might, for example, explore using it to help you respond to a range of situations, not only serious adversity but also the many more mundane challenges we face in our daily lives.

Self-talk for the flexibility sequence takes a different form. The flexibility sequence is composed of specific behaviors, not beliefs, and involves cycling through these behaviors in serial order. Thus, self-talk for the sequence becomes a process of inquiry. It is less a motivational monologue and more of an internal *dialogue* in which we pose questions to ourselves.[14] I mentioned some of these questions earlier, when we discussed how Paul used the sequence. When we apply the technique intentionally, and think about the nature of our contextual demands and how we might best respond to them, we mentally ask ourselves, for example, "What is happening?" and "What do I need to do?" How we answer these questions will depend on whatever resources or strategies we have in our repertoire, which leads us to ask, "What am I able to do?" And, finally, as we observe the outcome of these decisions, and begin to plan our next steps, we ask ourselves, "Is it working?"

Like the self-talk statements of the mindset, the self-talk questions of the sequence can serve as reminders that we can try out, and use, different behaviors. Asking such questions can help us to practice and cultivate these abilities. Practice can be particularly helpful if there is a specific step in the sequence that we find especially difficult. Our research has shown that while most people are reasonably able to engage in each step of the sequence, some people do struggle with specific steps. In this case, paying particular attention to self-talk for a step that we find difficult could be useful in ameliorating that deficit.

Self-talk questions also serve the more global function of reminding us that the flexibility sequence is in fact a sequence. And for that sequence to be effective, we need to coordinate the different component skills, track how we are doing, and adjust or change as we go along. Asking ourselves self-talk questions with the sequence in mind helps to guide us through the steps.

To make all of this a bit easier for those who wish to practice or explore this kind of self-talk on their own, I've listed examples for both the flexibility mindset and the flexibility sequence in the accompanying figure. I've included alternatives so that you can choose the versions that best suit your personal preferences.

237

Flexibility Mindset	Self-talk statements	Distanced self-talk statements	Alternative self-talk statements
Optimism	The future will be okay.	[Your name], the future will be okay.	This will pass. It may not turn out exactly as I want it to, but I will be fine. Everything will work out. Life will go on and it will be fine.
Confidence in coping	I have the skills.	[Your name] has the skills. [Your name], you have the skills.	I can do it. I can cope with this. I can handle it. I can solve most problems. I can usually find a solution.
Challenge appraisal	I will do what is necessary.	[Your name] will do what is necessary. [Your name], you will do what is necessary.	I will do my best. I am up to the challenge. I will work it out. I will get past this.

Flexibility Sequence	Self-talk questions	Distanced self-talk questions	Alternative self-talk questions
Context sensitivity	What is happening? What do I need to do?	[Your name], what is happening? What does [your name] need to do? [Your name], what do you need to do?	Why am I feeling this way? What would solve the problem? How can I change this?
Repertoire	What am I able to do?	What is [your name] able to do? [Your name], what are you able to do?	What strategies do I know how to use? What resources do I have at my disposal?
Feedback monitoring	Is it working?	[Your name], is it working?	Did I solve problem? Am I making progress? Do I feel better? Should I modify how I am doing this? Should I try something else? Can I use a new strategy?

Figure 5.

Some of these choices employ the common technique of inserting second-person pronouns or even your own name into these phrases. This kind of self-talk is known as distanced self-talk. If I did this with my own name, for example, instead of saying, "I have the skills to get the job done," I would say, "George has the skills to get the job done," or, "George, you have the skills to get the job done." Instead of asking myself, "What am I able to do?" I would ask, "What is George able to do?" or, "George, what are you able to do?" Although it might seem a bit odd to speak of yourself this way, the research of psychologist Ethan Kross has shown distanced self-talk to be especially effective for dealing with emotional situations. The reason is that second-person language provides some psychological distance, as if you are observing or talking to yourself from afar, and that distance makes it a bit easier to reframe the meaning of whatever is going on at the time. If you remember, Paul used distanced self-talk to help break out of his emotional rut and shift his thinking toward a flexibility mindset. ("C'mon Paul," he told himself, "get a grip. You can get past this. You're a smart guy. You can figure it out.")[15]

The key to all these self-talk variants, as has been the case with most of what we've discussed in this book, is that it is not so much what you do but that what you do actually works. And in this spirit, you can explore each of these different forms of self-talk as it suits your needs. Or you can create your own self-talk.

A Bright Light Barely Visible

When we last checked on Jed, he was in serious trouble. The cerebrospinal fluid leak had really thrown him, and nothing he was trying seemed to be helping him regain his equilibrium. He was out of options.

Apart from the sheer emotional pain of what he was experiencing, his downward-spiraling mood began to chip away at the flexibility mindset he had relied upon for so long. The sheer weight of this new round of disappointments, heaped on everything else he'd already been through, began to feel like it was smothering him. It was like throwing a blanket on a bright light. The light still peeked through, but it was now barely visible. Of course, he could still try to think his way through the flexibility sequence. He knew what he could do. But without the motivational thrust of that optimistic, confident, challenge-oriented mindset propelling him forward, it was going to be that much harder.

The Future Will Be Okay. I Have the Skills.
I Will Do What Is Necessary.

Jed never gave up. His light had dimmed, but it hadn't completely gone out. He kept struggling and eventually he struggled his way back. He was able to do this in part by spontaneously developing his own version of self-talk to gradually rekindle a flexibility mindset. Little by little, he reframed his frustrating experiences as incremental improvements.

"My sister was really helpful in this way," he said. "She would say, like, 'Dude, I know this is bad, but you know you've got this doctor's appointment coming up, and then there is going to be this other thing.' I would talk it out with her. And she would give me that check for the, whatever you could call it, cognitive distortion. She would help me see my own progress.

"Thoughts like, 'This might not get better,' were really bad. But other thoughts, 'This could get better,' or 'This is getting better,' or 'This is already better than it was,' these thoughts helped keep me buoyant. I don't know how conscious I was of doing it. You know, I didn't say to myself, 'Oh, I have to reframe this.' But when I was in that state, not knowing how long it was going to last, and just feeling awful, you know, thinking, 'Is this going to persist?' was a really depressing thought. But if I thought, 'This is bad now, but there is hope for the future,' you know, it was like I was marking progress for myself."

What Is Happening? What Do I Need to Do?

After the accident and the amputation, Jed had adapted by using the tools and resources he knew best. This new challenge threw him. The demands were profoundly different, and far more cryptic. Although he had used the flexibility sequence previously, he was barely aware of having done so. When this new challenge hit, he was forced by circumstance to think it through, to learn more explicitly how he had coped so well in the past. For instance, he became exquisitely sensitized to the shifting contextual demands that now confronted him. And as his growing sensitivity to the changes in his world sharpened, his insights about the changes became crystal clear.

As he remembers it, "When I think about recovering from the accident, there are two things that stand out: one, the problem was clear, and two, it didn't affect my cognition, my ability to think, in any demonstrable way, you know, nothing from the chest up. Except for the pain, which was always distressing. Over the long run, there were good times and bad times, but, overall, I could see I was getting better. With this new one [the CSF leak], it was unclear what was happening, and what the treatment was. I saw all kinds of specialists. I was lying down in their offices trying to figure out what the hell was going on, what to do. They all said something different. Some doctors said do surgery right away. Other doctors said, no, wait. And I was in this fog, you know, my head was so fuzzy all the time, and my daily experience, it was profoundly troubling, you know, any time I moved around."

What Am I Able to Do?

One of the hardest insights for Jed was the realization that he could no longer rely on what had been the most effective tool in his repertoire, his network of social support.

"In some ways, my questions about why didn't I have trauma symptoms [after the accident] were answered by social support. There was just this huge swell of people from the restaurant, and all of our friends and different groups of people just swooped in around us and carried us through that whole thing. I just thought that was the biggest thing. But with this one [the CSF leak], the big problem was I just didn't feel like myself.

"I tried engaging with people, but I couldn't, partly because I just felt like shit. I didn't want to have to pretend. I mean, there was some of that burden in the hospital, after the accident, like when people would come by. And I would have to put my best foot forward. It was kind of exhausting. But I was capable of doing it, and there was some reciprocity in that process. I also felt, you know, obligated because people had been so good to me, and it felt like a pure, you know, relationship thing. But this new one, it felt like the only thing I could do was limit my mobility and activity to mitigate some of the symptoms, and when people came over I didn't really feel capable of engaging. My thoughts were disoriented. I felt foggy, you know, cognitively foggy."

It's difficult to imagine that support from other people wouldn't always be a plus. Humans are social creatures. We constantly rely on others and we engage in cooperative behavior to an extraordinary level. When we are around people we care about, people we feel some attachment or bond with, cooperation goes much further. We tend to give more, and we tend to expect more in return. And when we need help, or just a shoulder to cry on, we know we can usually count on at least some of those close to us to provide it.

Not surprisingly, social support, as this aspect of human behavior is known, is a solid predictor of resilient outcomes. Across studies, actually, it's probably the most consistent predictor. But, as we've now seen many times, the size of the effects—how much social support actually tells us overall about the likelihood that a person will be resilient—is typically small. That's because, as we've also now seen many times, it is not always effective. Interactions with friends and relatives are sometimes even harmful. And sometimes our pain can drive away supports. When people are struggling for a long period of time, well-intending friends or relatives may become frustrated, or find the constant negative emotion so taxing that they gradually pull away.[16]

Jed was acutely aware of these possibilities. He knew there needed to be at least some reciprocity in social interactions, even relatively one-directional support-giving interactions. With this latest round of difficulties, he found he simply wasn't up to it. He also knew that he had been relying heavily on his support network for a long time, ever since the accident. Then the need had lifted somewhat, and it seemed like a lot to ask people to go back in that direction. As he put it, "I didn't want to initiate compassion fatigue in my social circle."

I experienced Jed's gradual pulling away firsthand. During the course of our work together, we had developed a close mentor-student bond. In many ways it had also become a solid friendship. I have always socialized with my students. It is not uncommon for my entire lab to share meals or drinks together, or occasionally to attend concerts around the city. I had an extra-special relationship with Jed, however, because I deeply respected him, both for surviving what he had survived and because of how, despite all he'd been through, he was still able to engage with other people on a very human level. The pain of those previous years had not jaded him. He was not bitter. It seemed that he was even more enduringly warm and approachable *because* of what he'd been through. That generosity of spirit made Jed the kind of person other people wanted to give back to. As his mentor and friend, I felt this deeply. But in this latest crisis, it seemed pretty clear that Jed was not looking for support from the world around him, including me. If anything, he was shunning it. He retreated, almost unnoticeably at first, but then eventually it became literally impossible for me or anyone else from the lab to visit him or even correspond by email. It was as if the fog in his head had extended to a veil of fog around him. At some point it became obvious, without Jed ever saying it, that he needed it to be that way.

Is It Working?

What truly seemed to have saved Jed, what got him through this new part of the crisis, was his ability to regroup using the feedback monitoring step. He had clarified for himself the new challenge ("I just didn't feel like myself"). He knew that one of the best tools he had, his network of supports, wasn't helping him anymore ("I didn't want to interact with other people"). And he found other ways to get by. He learned, for example, that he could still find succor if he narrowed the scope of his social network to his core family.

"It felt like an incubation. You know, like I wrapped myself up. My mental state was so contingent on my bodily state. And the only way for my body to get through this was to cocoon with Meg and our kids. They became my whole life. That was the sphere. We had just moved into student housing. This tiny little boxy apartment. It was much smaller than where we had been before. My brother-in-law and his crew moved us in, because I was in the hospital and Megan was at her wit's end. Megan was literally handling everything.

"I tried to be active, to get my mind off the symptoms. You know, just to be engaged with things. But I mean I couldn't be active. That was the crazy thing. Every time I stood up or even sat up, the symptoms came back immediately.

"I spent a good deal of time during the first few months with my newborn son sleeping on my chest. For naps, you know. I had him in this thing and I would shake him a bit, rock him, and we would nap together."

The dizziness and cognitive fog made anything that took much effort extremely difficult. Steady mental work or concentration was nearly impossible.

"I tried reading. That was really hard."

Distraction became crucial for Jed.

"I think that was when I discovered playing video games on my phone, as a distraction. I was just trying to keep myself mentally on track. The passivity of, you know, just having something like entertainment was easier. At first, I was actually playing the video games on my phone. Then I started watching people play video games. This was like a hobby I took up. I am kind of ashamed about it [laughs]."

Puzzled, I asked Jed how he was able to watch people play video games.

"Twitch," he told me, and when he saw my blank expression, he shot back with a broad, almost teasing smile, "You don't know about Twitch?"

Jed explained that Twitch is an online platform that allows gamers to stream their games in real time for anyone to watch.

"It's been the biggest thing. Like the new radio DJ. Someone has this personality, and then twenty thousand people tune in to watch them play video games. Everybody is typing. So, there's this ongoing streaming, typing, and chatting. It's a whole thing. So I started doing that. It was pure distraction. That was probably the best thing I found. I mean the most specific relief I could get was to completely distract myself. Something like that, lying down watching video games, or a movie.

"So, I had these things, distraction and being around my family. Megan was incredible. Just incredible. That would send me to tears. You know, she just, that woman is a soldier. She never gave me a hard time. Of course, there were times when she just reached a breaking point, where she was like, this thing is never going to get better, and she didn't know what the hell she had gotten into with two kids and a guy who can't get out of bed, but that's a crazy prospect to be in that situation. It was like we wiggled our way through it, and I would, you know, gradually make improvements. But it was two years, two whole years when it was really bad."

Jed also found that he had a few other tools up his sleeve.

"There was a lot of levity, if I think back. There was love for my daughter. She was fun. She is such a lively, energetic person. She's got this acerbic wit. And I did what I could with the kids. You know, my son was a baby at the time, so I did diaper changes. There is a lot you can actually do from a bed."

The New Normal

Jed saw some improvement, but it was always fleeting. Whatever progress he made came in fits and starts, and it was frustratingly inconsistent. Sometime in February, his doctors tried an epidural blood patch. This was by no means a simple procedure. The patient's blood is removed and then injected into the epidural space surrounding the spine just below the site of the CSF leak. There are always risks in any surgical procedure involving the spine, as attested to by Jed's ongoing difficulties. But this procedure was actually successful and afforded noticeable improvement in his symptoms. Unfortunately, the gains never lasted long. Jed tried a second procedure and then a third. Each time the story was the same, short-term improvement followed by backsliding to more or less the same place.

By the end of the year, genuine recovery seemed as far off as ever. Jed was beginning to feel desperate.

"I was pretty much at my wit's end. After everything we tried, I was stuck again in bed, not doing well, with lots of severe headaches."

It was especially painful for him to think about his larger goals.

"I had to kind of jettison the long-term concrete goals of getting better and finally achieving the PhD. Those two goals began to feel out of reach. It was painful. The PhD was really painful. I had missed interviews, so I was already a year behind. I was in the same externship, and I hadn't made any demonstrative progress. I couldn't work on my projects, intellectually. It was always fits and starts."

It was then that Jed began consulting with a well-known spinal neurosurgeon on the West Coast. A cyst had developed along Jed's spine at the site of the leakage. The West Coast neurosurgeon had been using an extensive surgical procedure that could remove it. It was risky, of course, riskier than the epidural patch. It would also mean an exhausting flight across the country. Seeing no other options, in the spring of that year Jed made the trip. It turned out to be one of the most difficult experiences of his long and painful saga.

"The postsurgical recovery was brutal. The worst headaches yet. What I thought was my pain threshold just kept getting louder and louder. When I woke up from that surgery, my whole head was like 'whomp . . . whomp . . . whomp. . . .' So crazy painful. They gave me opioids, or whatever they give you after surgery. That just numbed me out a bit. Not much more."

The surgery was successful in removing the cyst, but unfortunately, not much else. Most of Jed's symptoms remained. Some were even worse, especially the headaches.

The disappointment was overwhelming.

"You know, it's something I didn't bargain for, something that, you know, affects brain functioning. And even the prospect that this could be a permanent thing that just fucking happened, that's going to be with me forever, I was not even able to entertain that. I wasn't even considering that for a long time."

What Is Happening? What Do I Need to Do?

Jed had come to a crossroads. There wasn't much else left he could try, and, with this latest setback, that reality was staring him down. It was agonizing. But, as he reflected on his prospects, he began to come to terms with the fact that the challenge had shifted.

"I think it was maybe in the summer. There was this period of transition. It started to feel like, 'Okay, I've had most of the interventions that they can offer me.' Nothing really worked. I still didn't know why I had residual symptoms. There was going to have to be a turning point. I had to come to terms with it. I had to accept that this was the new normal. This is like, 'I am going to have, for the foreseeable future, this set of symptoms which are demonstrably worse than everything that came before, even the accident, because they affect my ability to focus and work and think.'"

Jed's reflections, as wrenching as they were, led him to a profound insight. Not exactly the kind of bolt-from-the-blue epiphany that had propelled Paul out of his apartment. But there were parallels. Jed had progressively come to the realization that his new difficulties might be permanent, that there may very well be no fix. And if that was true, as much as he wished it otherwise, he had no choice but to accept where he was and go from there.

"There were really no other avenues to explore. So, like, I came to, whatever happens, this is what I've got now. This is my new baseline."

Jed's insight was the product of an almost aching sensitivity to context. And fueled by the realization it brought him, he began to rethink the challenge. He made a conscious decision. He was going to have to stop focusing on how bad his symptoms were, on finding a "cure," because, in all likelihood, there wasn't going to be one. Instead, he would have to concentrate on finding better ways to manage his symptoms. He would shift his energy to trying to improve whatever he could.

What Am I Able to Do?

Jed had already assessed the new challenge. He knew what he had to do. His previous ordeals had also given him a pretty good idea of his repertoire. He knew what worked. But this new challenge he was facing was clearly different. He had never encountered anything like it before. It was vague and debilitating, with no clear cause. But even more than that, it wouldn't go away. As Jed summarized it, "You know, there's like this event that's not in the past. It's here, and it just keeps on cycling forward." It became increasingly obvious to Jed that he was going to have to explore using new strategies to deal with the ongoing problem.

Is It Working?

Jed tried whatever he could think of that might help him manage his symptoms, and then he monitored the effects. If a strategy was helpful, he added it to his repertoire. If not, he either discarded it or readjusted and tried again.

One approach he explored was pushing himself back out into the world as best he could manage. He planned to take it slowly at first and then, if all went well, gradually pick up the pace. He knew it was going to be an enormously difficult road, with plenty of ups and downs. But he made gains, and, slowly, he was able to turn his life back toward something that had begun to feel almost normal.

He didn't need to jettison everything that had worked for him in the past. In fact, one of the biggest bonuses that came with his gradual return to the external world, he discovered, was that he could again seek the comfort of his support network. His family life grew steadier, and he was slowly able to move around more easily and take on more responsibilities. His social world expanded back outward. And slowly, it was possible to have friends around again and to enjoy their company and support.

Jed had also learned to pace himself. He began planning rest periods, ways he could recharge at the end of the day or when he was free of obligations. As he resumed more concentrated social interactions with family and friends, he discovered that it was enormously helpful to excuse himself for short periods of time, say fifteen minutes, to find a quiet room where he could lie down and dim the pain.

He experimented with exercise as well. At first, this was an abysmal failure. Any kind of intense exercise only made the symptoms worse. Then he discovered that short stints on a stationary bicycle were possible, and gradually, in increments, he increased these to last longer. He built up his stamina, and over time exercise became an indispensable means of boosting his mood. He also sometimes used mindfulness meditation as a way to keep his perspective, along with breathing exercises to help relax his body. These techniques weren't always helpful, but through trial and error Jed learned when they were most effective.

Jed got some unexpected support when he discovered a neurologist who specialized in the same cluster of symptoms he had been struggling with. She reaffirmed his approach, which was a great confidence boost, and furnished him with even more techniques to help manage the symptoms, in particular the searing intensity of the headache pain. By this point, Jed knew that not everything would work. He cycled through each of the new techniques she had suggested, applying the same trial-and-error method he had already been using. Anything that was helpful, he added to his growing repertoire.

Cycling Forward

Jed was making genuine progress. For the past several years, symptoms and treatments had cycled in and out of his life. It was literally dizzying. Now he had begun to gain control. Now it was Jed, and not his maladies, that was cycling forward.

He began to have "pockets of good days, when the headaches weren't disabling," and he used these small respites to inch himself closer to his former external life. At one point, he rejoined my research lab. Sometimes he would simply hang out for a bit, or work in one of the small rooms in the back of the lab. He began attending meetings with us, initially only sporadically, and then more regularly. On occasion, when he was up to it, we would chat, catching up on work and life, even laughing, just as we had before his setback.

As he acclimated further, Jed was able to resume work on some of the research projects he had been involved in, and as his physical presence in the lab increased, we were able to return to regular discussions about a manuscript we had put aside two years earlier. Jed's progress was slow but steady, and eventually, against all odds, he completed the manuscript. Several months later we got the wonderful news that it had been accepted for publication. This was a huge milestone for Jed, and it was another decisive affirmation of his efforts.

He reached an even bigger milestone when he was able to resume his duties on a clinical externship he had started two years earlier. He still missed days occasionally, when the symptoms became unbearable, but thanks to the patience of the externship staff, he eventually completed the rotation. Then he began another, even more demanding externship, this time in neuropsychology. The rotation required two full days a week. It was a lot, and there were times when he could barely manage. "By the time five o'clock rolled around, after a full day, my head was like bursting. I could barely even think. I just had these blazing, blazing headaches," he said. But increasingly, with the tools he had acquired, he was able to endure longer and longer stretches. And, impressively, he was able to complete that externship too.

"I can't remember all of this precisely, but man, it was huge. It was a big thing, just being active, and involved. I can't tell you. I had been, you know, getting kind of funky. My mood. When I got myself back out there, my mood changed right away. It kind of set my head right, put me back on track. I felt like I could be myself again. I could be effective again."

CHAPTER 10

And Then There Was a Global Pandemic

I n the fall of 2019, in the midst of writing this book, I began planning a springtime sabbatical trip to Europe. The idea was to travel by train, writing and giving lectures along the way. My wife, Paulette, would join me. She would also be working on a book project.

As I was making these plans, a few people in Wuhan, China, started experiencing some strange symptoms. By late December, Jinyintan Hospital had reported several patients suffering from a pneumonia-like illness of unknown origin.[1] The illness was eventually given a name, 2019-nCoV. At the time, it didn't seem like anything to worry about, at least not in New York or Europe. Then it began to spread and was given a new name, SARS-CoV-2.

That name got my attention. I had done research on survivors of the SARS epidemic in Hong Kong back in 2003. SARS was a brutal virus that produced a dangerously high mortality rate. Although most of its impact was felt in Asia, it managed to spread itself around the globe before it was finally contained.[2]

Not much was yet known about this new variant of SARS, but when cases appeared outside of China and its spread picked up speed, the world took notice. By late January 2020, the World Health Organization had declared a global health emergency. The virus got another new name, COVID-19. By late February, it had already exceeded the original SARS virus in both confirmed cases and virus-related deaths.[3] Soon cases were being reported in the Lombardy region of Italy, one of the destinations on my travel itinerary. It seemed to be spreading rapidly there, too.

Paulette and I were concerned, but, perhaps foolishly, we decided to go ahead with our trip. One of the lectures I was to deliver was at a World Health Organization (WHO) meeting in Geneva. The WHO had not yet canceled the meeting, which I took as a sign that perhaps the virus might be contained. Besides, Italy was the very last stop on our agenda. If the virus was still active by that time, we could always cancel that segment of the trip and return home a bit earlier.

We flew out on March 3. First stop, Bergen, Norway. Everything seemed more or less normal there. The virus was a topic of conversation, but there were no masks, and the term "social distancing" had not yet entered the lexicon. We had a nice little apartment on a quiet street in the old part of the city, near the university. It rained a lot. I was busy giving lectures, and in the evenings Paulette and I joined my colleagues for dinner. We found time over the weekend for a delightful boat tour of the nearby Modalen fjord.

But worry steadily crept in. Our son, twenty-two, was in New York by himself. We'd heard reports of the virus spreading in the United States and of food runs in grocery stores. Our daughter was still away at college, but then her college closed down. Still, these were seen as temporary measures. Colleges were not yet closing for the semester, only switching to online classes as a temporary fix until things calmed down.

A week later, we took the night train to Oslo. This was a bucket-list item for me. I love trains. Although we had a sleeper room, I stayed up most of the night, watching out the window as moonlit fields and snow-covered mountains appeared and disappeared. I was tired by morning, but had enough energy to deliver a lecture at the University of Oslo. Although my colleagues had warned me that the talk might not be very well attended because of the virus, the room was packed. There were still no visible signs of concern: no masks, no social-distancing efforts. Afterward I learned that the WHO had just declared the virus a global pandemic. The university was shifting gears and was now planning to close entirely the very next day. The news was discordant, hard to take in.

We were scheduled to travel the following morning to Copen-hagen. There had only been a few cases there, and we assumed we'd be able to assess the situation further when we arrived. In the middle of the night, I received a text from one of my Danish colleagues telling me not to come. The border was closing. Then we saw the headline that the United States was planning to bar air travel from Europe. The emergency had accelerated at what seemed like an im-plausible clip. We scrambled to get flights and barely made it back to New York in time.

•

VIRUSES ARE INGENIOUS little things. Although COVID-19 seemed like SARS, it spread differently. SARS was passed on from the lungs. People who were infected and seriously ill could transmit the virus by respiration. Early research showed that COVID-19 was spread-ing by respiration as well, but it didn't appear to have to wait until its host had showed symptoms. COVID-19 was able to spread almost immediately. This meant that literally anyone who came in contact with the virus, whether seriously ill or not, was a transmission vector.[4] This was how it was spreading so quickly. And back when the virus was still new, people without symptoms were almost completely unconcerned and took no measures to protect others from their exposure.

Life in New York City, when we returned, still bore a semblance of normality. We were required to self-isolate in our New York apartment for two weeks, because we had been in Europe. At the time, I thought this was a bit extreme. I watched with envy from my window as people went about their business. But case counts were already rising steeply, and by the time our quarantine had ended it no longer mattered. By then, the entire city was in lockdown.

It turned out that New York was a perfect breeding ground for the virus. Its large population was densely packed into a culturally and ethnically diverse city that is also the primary point of entry for air travel into the United States. Over one hundred million passengers use its airports annually, and, as tracking studies later showed, much of the virus's spread across the country stemmed from travel through New York.[5]

Only a few short weeks after our return, the daily numbers in New York had risen to shocking levels: over six thousand new cases, two thousand hospitalizations, and eight hundred deaths *per day*! The hospital down the street from my apartment closed off an entire block and set up a triage tent. A refrigerator truck was installed outside as a makeshift morgue. The same was happening all around the city. Hospitals were being overwhelmed, and soon temporary hospital tents would appear nearby in Central Park for the overflow.

•

AT THE TIME I am writing this, the pandemic is still ongoing. A vaccine rollout is in the early stages and a return to normalcy appears to be on the horizon, only it is not yet possible to pinpoint exactly when that will be. In the meantime, there is no choice but to continue dealing with the situation.

Throughout the pandemic, the key points of this book have been in full evidence.

Predictably, the resilience blind spot made an early appearance. As the case counts racked up, media outlets dutifully sounded the alarm. In early May 2020, one prominent newspaper reported that "federal agencies and experts warn that a historic wave of mental health problems is approaching: depression, substance abuse, post-traumatic stress disorder and suicide." The mental health system, the paper concluded, was not prepared to handle the coming surge. To back up that point, national polling data were cited showing that "nearly half of Americans report the coronavirus is harming their mental health."[6]

The pandemic was stressful, to be sure, but to my ear such dire forecasts were eerily reminiscent of the distorted expectations of widespread trauma following the 9/11 attacks. The national poll data, mentioned as evidence for the coming onslaught of psychological casualties, actually showed a more nuanced picture. Only 19 percent of Americans felt the coronavirus was having a major impact on their mental health, while the bulk of those polled, 81 percent, felt the virus had only a minor impact or no impact at all.[7] Nineteen percent was a lot of people—almost one in five—to have serious mental health concerns, but with the scale of the difficulties and the uncertainty wrought by the virus, wouldn't we expect as much?

Based on everything we've learned, it's pretty clear at this point that most people who are exposed to potentially traumatic events do experience at least some traumatic stress early on. That doesn't mean that everyone is traumatized or will develop PTSD. Rather, it shows that traumatic stress is a natural response to a highly challenging event. In accordance with these findings, COVID, for most people, was a source of ongoing fear. It caused difficulties and challenges.

And in that context, at least some anxious concern is to be expected. When presented with the polling data, Joshua Gordon, the director of the National Institute of Mental Health, put it this way: "Given the circumstances, feeling anxious is part of a normal response to what's going on."[8]

As we saw earlier in the book, most people confronted with a potentially traumatic event do not experience enduring trauma reactions. They are resilient. In other words, for most people, traumatic stress dissipates as they find ways to flexibly adapt to the challenges an event poses. We were seeing this, too, during the pandemic. As the crisis wore on, most people found ways to manage, and the anxiety or depression or stress they had been experiencing earlier began to fade.

By the same token, as always, the stress was not the same for everybody. Every aversive event is unique, and the COVID-19 pandemic was in many ways as varied and multifaceted as any event we are likely to face. It was difficult to categorize, especially in the beginning. Was it a trauma? A source of chronic stress? A depressing bereavement? A catastrophe waiting to happen? Even more complex, its consequences diverged dramatically for different people.

·

EARLY ON IN the crisis, the COVID pandemic was just about the only thing anyone talked about. Not surprisingly, given what I do for a living, fielding questions from journalists became a regular part of my daily routine. My typical refrain went something like this:

The key task for most people is to keep stress at a minimum. Everyone is adapting to a new reality that includes, in one form or another, fears about viral spread and contagion, the stress of self-quarantine, supply shortages, caring for loved ones, and uncertainty about the future. Some are also coping with illness and fear of death, fears about the health of loved ones, and looming financial losses. Overcoming these stresses and finding our way to resilience means reflecting on our own evolving situation and using whatever tools we already have at our disposal to manage it. In other words, we need to be flexible.[9]

It was not an easy sell. The spread of the virus was confusing and frightening, especially early on, and the catastrophic forecasts circulating in the media only amplified the sense of dread. The antidote I suggested to help people fight off the stress, as you may have already guessed, was a flexibility mindset. At every opportunity, I repeated the same mantra:

This pandemic is not easy, but we can manage it. We will get through it. Human beings have always shown abundant psychological resilience in the face of just about every imaginable adversity, and we will do it this time too.

It was equally critical to mention the resilience paradox. Predictably, news stories had already begun to appear touting the key traits of resilience. Although well-meaning, such advice is misleading and in the end not likely to be helpful. Instead, I stressed a different approach:

There is no "magic bullet," no single best way to cope for everyone. Every trait, every resource, every behavior, has both costs and benefits. What works in one situation for one person may not be effective for another person, or even for the same person in another situation or at another point in time.

And, of course, I emphasized solving this paradox with the flexibility sequence:

We need to pay attention to what is happening to us, adjust our behavior to fit whatever the situation is calling for, and monitor ourselves to make sure whatever we are doing is working. If it isn't, we need to switch to something else. And we need to keep doing this. Life doesn't sit still, and this pandemic won't either. We need to keep adjusting and readjusting as we go along.

.

Reina was resilient following her harrowing experience of the 9/11 attacks, but she found the COVID crisis unexpectedly difficult. In the years since 9/11, she had had her ups and downs. She remained in New York throughout that period, and she continued working and caring for her family as best she could. She was good at what she did, and her career flourished. Unfortunately, her marriage fell apart. Along the way, she also experienced some serious health issues that left her immune system compromised. Still, she kept her life more or less on track, even during these difficulties, and eventually she remarried. Although the path was not always easy, she felt she was in about as good a shape psychologically as she could have hoped for.

The COVID crisis threw her for a loop. A compromised immune system meant that she needed to be extra careful about inadvertent exposure to the virus. And as the lockdown in New York ramped up, she found herself feeling increasingly anxious. Eventually, it became unbearable, and she didn't know how to stop it. This was an unusual experience for Reina. She had always had a pretty well-articulated flexibility mindset. She was optimistic and confident and almost always found flexible solutions to the challenges she faced. The feeling of helplessness was new, and it confused her.

But Reina didn't give up. She held on to enough of a flexibility mindset to tell herself that she would eventually figure it out. Fittingly, she did find her way to a flexible solution. It was by trying something new, something she had never thought of doing before. She sought the help of a therapist.

This was Reina's version of coping ugly. She had never been particularly interested in psychotherapy and admitted to feeling somewhat disdainful about the process. But she needed help, and she was insightful enough to recognize it. At this point in the pandemic, it was no longer possible to visit a therapist's office. So she met and worked with her new therapist online. The therapist helped her parse out options. Reina learned new techniques to manage the anxiety, and as she did, her confidence and optimism were again bolstered.

In due course, Reina's therapist also helped her to realize that what she really wanted to do was to leave the city. Reina had always thought of herself as a die-hard New Yorker. Leaving the city seemed like a betrayal. Her therapist helped her to understand that she could leave as a temporary option. Her children had grown, and both she and her husband had jobs that allowed them to work remotely. The extra stress caused by her physical vulnerabilities was harming her. She needed a break. So why not take it?

Reina discussed the option with her husband, and they jointly decided to rent a house several hours from the city. Right away, it was clear that she had made the right choice, at least for this particular problem at this particular moment in her life. Whether or not they would remain out of the city was a question for another day. Reina was confident they would be able to work out that answer when the time came.

•

SOME STRATEGIES EMERGED as especially apt for coping with a pandemic lockdown. These included, for example, relying on the support of others; bonding with those close to us; keeping informed, but not overindulging in media consumption; using distractions; and finding ways to laugh or relax through activities such as watching movies or reading. It was especially important, as research had already begun to show, to minimize isolation by having joint family activities and by keeping in touch with friends and colleagues by phone or video chat, or whatever other means were available.

The key to using these strategies, as always, hinged on the steps of the flexibility sequence: assessing the contextual demands of the moment, applying a strategy from our own repertoire that might meet those demands, monitoring the result to check how well it is working, and then keeping it up or changing or adjusting it as necessary.

The sheer duration of the pandemic, in particular, cast a spotlight on the importance of staying motivated and engaged with a flexibility mindset and repeatedly cycling through the flexibility sequence. The pandemic seemed to be never-ending, and that meant a steady flow of situational demands. These demands were constantly changing. What worked best was not only different for each person in each situation, but could be different for the same person at different points in time as the pandemic progressed. Initially, for example, social connection and bonding seemed crucial for just about everybody. But with time, as families found themselves locked down in close quarters, it became clear that it was also necessary to find ways to ensure privacy and personal space for solitude or quiet reflection.

My family and I had our own challenges. First, my ninety-seven-year-old mother suffered a mild stroke and needed to be hospitalized. Her age put her at great risk, and that had us all deeply worried. Fortunately, no small thanks to the tireless efforts of my brothers, Fred and Alan, she remained virus-free, and after a few days she returned home safely. But then, in November 2020, as the second wave of the virus kicked in, both Fred and my mother tested positive for COVID. Fred had only mild symptoms, but my mother deteriorated rapidly. She had always been energetic and active, even in her nineties. The virus hit her so hard she could barely lift her head. As she was taken to the hospital by ambulance, we prepared ourselves for the worst.

The truly difficult part was that none of us were able to visit my mother. Even worse, due to her physical weakness and poor hearing, it was almost impossible to even speak with her over the phone. The lack of contact was excruciating, especially when we learned from the nursing staff that my mother seemed to be giving up. She was disoriented and withdrawn, and it was heartbreaking to think of her in that state, alone in her hospital bed with no one to comfort or reassure her.

But my brothers didn't rest. With no prompting from me—I learned long ago to keep my psychology background out of family discussions—Fred set up regular conference calls so the three of us could problem-solve together and find flexible solutions. We spoke regularly with the hospital staff and discussed different ways we might communicate with our mother. We brainstormed strategies to bolster her sagging mood and to keep her hopeful and positive. And we shared with each other any new information we could find on the virus and its treatment.

There was room for optimism. Not long after arriving in the hospital, my mother was given an infusion of antibody-rich plasma. It seemed to help her. Then, several days later, she received a new medication, remdesivir, that had just been approved by the FDA. Clinical trials had shown that the drug effectively reduced both recovery time and mortality. We hoped it would give my mother the boost she needed to pull through.

And then, against all odds, her health stabilized. Her spirits also began to improve. Several weeks later she was transferred to a COVID rehabilitation unit, and a bit after that, in what seemed like a miracle, she was given the all-clear to return home. We didn't yet know if there would be any lasting consequences from her bout with the virus. At her age, anything was possible. But the important thing, the very best thing, was that she was back in her own house, as she had so badly desired, and we were able to be with her again.

•

THROUGHOUT THE PANDEMIC, my go-to strategy for keeping myself balanced and on track was exercise. Intense aerobic runs and long walks in the park got me outside, kept me healthy, and cleared my mind. But then, in another unexpected turn of events, I needed to be hospitalized, not once but twice. The first was a planned surgery, the second an emergency appendectomy. Although neither hospitalization was directly related to COVID-19, it was nerve-wracking all the same to be in a crowded hospital during a global disease pandemic. But the biggest challenge for me was not the surgeries. Rather, it was the fact that I could no longer exercise during the recovery periods. While healing from the operations, I could barely walk, let alone run or jump. My own advice was again staring me in the face—I needed to be flexible—and I heeded it. I assessed the contextual demands, worked out alternative strategies to reduce the stress and keep myself on track, and then monitored how well they worked. And I got by.

.

WHILE PONDERING INJURIES and hospitalization in the context of the pandemic, I was reminded of Maren. During the course of recovering from her spinal cord injury, Maren was never overwhelmed by traumatic stress. Nor did she ever become deeply depressed or anxious. There were a few moments here and there, of course, but for the most part she kept herself on an even keel. She was focused on the challenge. She was optimistic, confident, and continually flexible in finding solutions. It was pretty clear that Maren was resilient.

When I suggested this to her, she readily agreed.

"Yes, it's true. I think it's all true."

And yet, she was humble about her achievements. She hastened to add, "It would be inaccurate to say that I *never* had any periods where I felt anxious or depressed."

But Maren was not referring to those first few years of recovery after the injury, when traumatic stress or depression would have seemed like a natural response. Then she was resolute and focused. Nothing was going to get in her way. Rather, she was describing the later periods, after she had regained the ability to walk, and then returned to Cambridge to finish her studies. Back in school, she had to confront the normal stresses of a full life, but now with the added burden of lingering disability and pain.

Maren never fully regained control of her right leg. To this day, her gait is unstable and she walks with a limp. Simple actions most of us take for granted, such as strolling a few blocks or climbing a single flight of stairs, for Maren can be exhausting enterprises. Yet, ever the optimistic problem-solver, she continues to strive for flexible solutions so that she can do more with her life. Her difficulty walking long distances, for example, led her to the discovery that she could get around more easily riding a bicycle or a kick scooter, which not only gave her greater mobility but also helped further strengthen her body.

After finishing her education at Cambridge, Maren moved to the United States to study for a PhD in clinical psychology. She married and several years ago gave birth to a beautiful girl, Ana Sofia. She is now a tenured professor and clinician. By any account she is living a full and enviable life. Yet each of these achievements has demanded a little extra push, a bit more effort than would be required of other people. Maren is resilient, but she is not superhuman. At times she has been overwhelmed by the weight of all she has set out for herself to accomplish. But still she keeps on.

When the COVID pandemic hit, Maren did what everyone else did. She adapted. Many of the challenges she faced were more or less the same challenges other people faced. Staying safe. Maintaining her career while home-schooling a child. Keeping in touch with friends and family, in whatever form possible. Trying to stay afloat financially.

But Maren also has her own particular physical challenges to contend with. I wondered if perhaps these might have made the COVID crisis extra difficult for her. When I asked her about this, her optimism and flexible resourcefulness immediately sparkled through.

"I actually haven't experienced the pandemic as more difficult for me than other people. To the contrary, I think that in some ways, the seven months I spent in inpatient rehabilitation [after the injury] made me feel confident that I could handle staying home during a lockdown. During the rehabilitation stay, I always kept myself busy, working out, doing all kinds of treatments, phone calls, reading, listening to audiobooks, having visitors, and talking to other patients."

The required self-isolation during the pandemic was for Maren simply another version of this same challenge.

"During the lockdown, I spent a lot of time doing little projects with Ana Sofia. For example, we created an indoor garden and wrote each other little notes. I've had so many beautiful moments with her during lockdown and throughout the summer."

And when there was stress, she found ways to deal with that, too.

"For some reason, the building I live in kept the pool open during that time and I went swimming every day, sometimes even twice a day. That was super helpful as a stress relief!"

•

FOR JED, THE pandemic was yet another roadblock in an endless series of roadblocks. Just prior to the onset of COVID, he had begun a one-year clinical internship in a rehabilitation hospital. The internship was a final requirement for his PhD. It was full-time and it was demanding. But he was managing. Then the pandemic threw everything into disorder. Like many, he began working from home. He shifted his appointments with patients to an online format. The change was disorienting, and taxing in new ways, but again he adapted.

I knew Jed had begun the internship. I knew he had still not fully recovered physically, that he still had symptoms. I asked him about it. "Yeah, it's better, but it's still with me," he told me. "In fact, I have a searing headache right now."

Yet, as always, he was taking it in stride. "It's all been part of learning to live with it."

That process, "learning to live with it," had taught Jed a great deal.

When he first began studying for a master's degree, years earlier, before the accident, he had read articles in the trauma literature on the importance of finding meaning. He tried it. He wrote down his ideas about God and the universe. He made it fit.

But the accident and all the enduring struggles that followed changed everything. Jed reinvented himself.

"I had to throw that out, chuck it. I did that willingly. It was a conscious thing, like 'I can't think that way anymore.' I reordered my sense of causality. You know, 'Bad things happen.' I reordered my worldview and replaced it with love of family and people, and service, you know, dedication to the field, science and career, being useful."

As his life stabilized, he found a way to honor that worldview in the work he did—and still does—with survivors of traumatic injuries. He'd been drawn to this area because of his own firsthand experiences. Still, initially he was tentative. Did he really want to go down this road? With time, he discovered a satisfying balance. His duties at the rehabilitation hospital afforded him opportunities to continue engaging in research and scholarship, which he found intellectually fulfilling, but also provided him the chance to give back, to be of service to others. Most important, Jed was good at it. In particular, he discovered that his own experiences provided him with unique inroads to the struggles his patients were going through.

"I repurposed it. It's almost like alcoholics sponsoring other alcoholics in AA. Like that model. I found a way to use my experience."

To illustrate the point, Jed told me a story. Earlier in his training, before COVID, a new patient had come on the unit. The patient was visibly stressed, tearful, having difficulties adjusting emotionally to the reality of his injury. Jed's supervisor mentioned that the therapist who had been working with this patient was currently away on vacation. The patient badly needed to talk to someone. He asked if Jed wouldn't mind checking in on him.

Jed, on crutches, ambled into the patient's room.

"There were a couple of niceties, and then he looked at me and he was like, 'Okay, I'll talk to you. This will be a fair fight.' I understood immediately what he meant. But just to make sure I got it, he repeated it a few times. Then he followed it up with, 'All these people [gestures broadly], they have me filling out questionnaires and whatever, I don't even read them. These people, they haven't lost anything.'"

Jed had certainly lost a great deal. But, as he's told me many times, he's also gained a great deal. The long road from that fateful night of the accident—already ten years in the past by then—through the ups and downs of recovery, the gradual reconciliation, and even the COVID-19 pandemic, was for Jed an evolving process of reinventing himself and adapting to what was happening to him. Flexibility was a big part of that process.

In the beginning, he was only vaguely aware of how he had managed to cope so well. He had no idea he was utilizing a flexibility mindset, or engaging in anything remotely like the flexibility sequence. Indeed, he had not yet even heard of these concepts. The questions he had about his own resilience changed that. His ongoing physical struggles changed it even more. These experiences, as painful as they were, forced him to think hard about what had happened to him, what was continuing to happen to him, and how he could live with it.

Somewhere along the way, he figured it out. He began to see his own capacity, his own ability, to adapt flexibly. And he was increasingly able to apply that capacity—to utilize the tools he had and those he discovered along the way—more consciously, more deliberately, and more effectively. It helped that he was studying psychology, but I think most of his learning came from his own personal experiences. In that sense, Jed had no choice. Learning how flexibility worked and thinking it through, it seemed, was the only way he would survive. The only way he would come out on the other side. Although he still struggled, he had put his life back on track and was forging ahead. And he knew, from that point forward, that whatever happened next, he would always be able to find a way to come out on the other side.

Acknowledgments

I am forever in debt to the many brave individuals who have participated in my research or shared their experiences with me over the years, none more so than Jed McGiffin. I had no idea, back when I first met Jed, that his story would someday form the core of a book. I had no idea, either, that he would become such a big part of my life: first as a student, then as a collaborator, then as a deeply valued friend. My profound debt also extends to Maren Westphal, both for her friendship and for her continual openness in talking about her experiences. Although I cannot thank the other individuals whose stories I've told by name, because of the need to preserve their confidentiality, my debt and gratitude are no less for it. This book would simply not have been possible without them.

The ideas that form the core of the book have been percolating for years. Too many people to mention individually have in one way or another helped to shepherd them into their present form. They include, first and foremost, my dear friend and collaborator Isaac Galatzer-Levy, who is always at the forefront with his intelligence, his generous soul, and his unfailing willingness to "hang" for a probing discussion. Thanks also to Jim Levine, my literary agent, for believing in this book and helping me whip the original proposal into shape, and to my wonderful editor at Basic Books, Eric Henney, for his friendly but razor-sharp and perfectly spot-on editorial insights. Eric's editorial guidance was valuable initially and then, as I worked through the final drafts, became indispensable. In that same vein, I would be remiss if I did not thank Katherine Streckfus for her impeccable copyediting and for her insightful suggestions that often went well beyond copyediting. Then, of course, there is my brilliant wife, Paulette Roberts, and my now adult children, Raphael and Angie, with whom I have shared a seemingly limitless stream of thought-provoking conversations. I would also like to thank Richard McNally for his fearless scholarship and wide-ranging book recommendations; Lisa Feldman Barrett for her friendship and all-around awesome mind; Dan Gilbert for offering support and encouragement when I most needed it; Matteo Malgaroli for his intelligence, wit, and priceless humor; Wendy Lichtenthal for the many discussions we've shared and for her always brilliant clinical insights; Dacher Keltner for his years of friendship and his ever-readiness to engage whatever question I might happen to throw at him; and David O'Connor for his generosity in supporting my research and for the baseball games.

So many other friends and colleagues have allowed me access to their inspiring minds: Amelia Aldao, Chris Brewin, Richard Bryant, Christine Cha, Bernard Chang, Cecilia Cheng, Jim Coan, Tracy Dennis-Tiwary, Carrie Donoho, Donald Edmundson, Iris Engelhard, Chris Fagundes, Barbara Fredrickson, Sandro Galea, James Gross, John Jost, Krys Kaniasty, Paul Kennedy, Ann Kring, Annette LaGreca, Einat Levy-Gigi, Peter Lude, Joshua Mailman, Douglas Mennin, Judy Moskowitz, Jennie Noll, Anthony Ong, Ruth Pat-Horenczyk, Bennett Porter, Dave Sbarra, Noam Schneck, Gal Sheppes, Tyler Smith, Lena Verdeli, Patricia Watson, and Seymour Weingarten, as well as, unfortunately, some who have passed on: Susan Folkman, Scott Lilienfeld, Walter Mischel, and Susan Nolen-Hoeksema.

I am forever thankful to the ever-changing cast of students, post-docs, and visiting scholars who have helped make my lab, the Loss, Trauma, and Emotion Lab at Teachers College, Columbia University, a thriving crucible for new ideas and critical thinking. Special thanks in relation to the concepts developed in this book go to Rohini Bagrodia, Jeff Birk, Charles Burton, Shuquan Chen, Karin Coifman, Philippa Connolly, Erica Diminich, Sumati Gupta, Ann-Christin Haag, Roland Hart, Wai Kai Hou, Sandy Huang, Kathleen Lalande, Kan Long, Jenny Lotterman, Marie Lundorff, Fiona Maccallum, Anthony Mancini, Laura Meli, Meaghan Mobbs, Tony Papa, Charlotte Pfeffer, Katharina Schultebraucks, and Zhuoying Zhu. And last but by no means least, thanks to my wonderful colleagues and collaborators in Italy: Vitorio Lenzo, Antonio Malgaroli, Marina Quattropani, and Emanuela Saita.

Notes

Introduction: Why Was I Doing Okay?

1. These anecdotes were submitted online in response to David Biello, "What Is a Medically Induced Coma and Why Is It Used?," *Scientific American*, January 10, 2011, www.scientificamerican.com/article/what-is-a-medically-induced-coma.

2. D. M. Wade, C. R. Brewin, D. C. J. Howell, E. White, M. G. Mythen, and J. A. Weinman, "Intrusive Memories of Hallucinations and Delusions in Traumatized Intensive Care Patients: An Interview Study," *British Journal of Health Psychology* 20, no. 3 (2015): 613–631, https://doi.org/10.1111/bjhp.12109.

3. Susan A. Gelman, *The Essential Child: Origins of Essentialism in Everyday Thought* (New York: Oxford University Press, 2003).

Chapter 1: The Invention of PTSD

1. Albert B. Lord, *The Singer of Tales* (Cambridge, MA: Harvard University Press, 1960).

2. Jonathan Shay, *Achilles in Vietnam: Combat Trauma and the Undoing of Character* (New York: Simon and Schuster, 1994).

3. Shay, *Achilles in Vietnam*.

4. Samuel Pepys, *The Diary of Samuel Pepys*, vol. 4, ed. Henry B. Wheatley (London: Bell and Sons, 1904 [1663]), 225.

5. Pepys, *Diary*, 4:190.

6. John Eric Erichsen, *On Railway and Other Injuries of the Nervous System* (Philadelphia: Henry C. Lea, 1867).

7. F. Lamprecht and M. Sack, "Posttraumatic Stress Disorder Revisited," *Psychosomatic Medicine* 64, no. 2 (2002): 222–237.

8. Hermann Oppenheim, *Die traumatischen Neurosen nach den in der Nervenklinik der Charité in den letzten 5 Jahren gesammelten Beobachtungen* (Berlin: Verlag von August Hirschwald, 1889). A second edition was published in 1892, and a third in 1918.

9. Richard Norton-Taylor, "Executed World War I Soldiers to Be Given Pardons," *Guardian*, August 15, 2006.

10. Norton-Taylor, "Executed World War I Soldiers."

11. Jon Stallworthy, *Wilfred Owen* (Oxford: Oxford University Press, 1974).

12. *The Great War and the Shaping of the 20th Century*, episode 5, "Mutiny," KCET Television/British Broadcasting Company, 1996.

13. Wilfred Owen, *Wilfred Owen: Complete Works*, Delphi Poets Series (Hastings, UK: Delphi Classics, 2012).

14. Owen, *Complete Works*.

15. S. N. Garfinkel, J. L. Abelson, A. P. King, R. K. Sripada, X. Wang, L. M. Gaines, and I. Liberzon, "Impaired Contextual Modulation of Memories in PTSD: An fMRI and Psychophysiological Study of Extinction Retention and Fear Renewal," *Journal of Neuroscience* 34, no. 40 (2014): 13435.

16. For an illuminating discussion of mental disorders versus medical diseases and how symptoms of the former develop, see R. J. McNally, "The Ontology of Posttraumatic Stress Disorder: Natural Kind, Social Construction, or Causal System?," *Clinical Psychology: Science and Practice* 19, no. 3 (2012): 220–228, https://doi.org/10.1111/cpsp.12001; R. J. McNally, D. J. Robinaugh, G. W. Y. Wu, L. Wang, M. K. Deserno, and D. Borsboom, "Mental Disorders as Causal Systems: A Network Approach to Posttraumatic Stress Disorder," *Clinical Psychological Science* 3, no. 6 (2015): 836–849, https://doi.org/10.1177/2167702614553230; D. Borsboom and A. O. J. Cramer, "Network Analysis: An Integrative Approach to the Structure of Psychopathology," *Annual Review of Clinical Psychology* 9 (2013): 91–121; D. Borsboom, A. O. J. Cramer, and A. Kalis, "Reductionism in Retreat," *Behavioral and Brain Sciences* 42 (2019): e32.

17. For examples of this problem with the PTSD diagnosis, see J. J. Broman-Fulks, K. J. Ruggiero, B. A. Green, D. W. Smith, R. F. Hanson, D. G. Kilpatrick, and B. E. Saunders, "The Latent Structure of Posttraumatic Stress Disorder Among Adolescents," *Journal of Traumatic Stress* 22, no. 2 (2009): 146–152, https://doi.org/10.1002/jts.20399; J. J. Broman-Fulks, K. J. Ruggiero, B. A. Green, D. G. Kilpatrick, C. K. Danielson, H. S. Resnick, and B. E. Saunders, "Taxometric Investigation of PTSD: Data from Two Nationally Representative Samples," *Behavior Therapy* 37, no. 4 (2006): 364–380, https://doi.org/10.1016/j.beth.2006.02.006. For broader models of the dimensional nature of mental disorders, see R. Kotov, C. J. Ruggero, R. F. Krueger, D. Watson, Q. Yuan, and M. Zimmerman, "New Dimensions in the Quantitative Classification of Mental Illness," *Archives of General Psychiatry* 68, no. 10 (2011): 1003–1011, https://doi.org/10.1001/archgenpsychiatry.2011.107; A. Caspi and T. Moffitt, "All for One and One for All: Mental Disorders in One Dimension," *American Journal of Psychiatry* 175, no. 9 (2018): 831–844, https://doi

.org/10.1176/appi.ajp.2018.17121383; C. C. Conway, M. K. Forbes, K. T. Forbush, E. I. Fried, M. N. Hallquist, R. Kotov, S. N. Mullins-Sweatt, et al., "A Hierarchical Taxonomy of Psychopathology Can Transform Mental Health Research," *Perspectives on Psychological Science* 14, no. 3 (2019): 419–436, https://doi.org/10.1177/1745691618810696.

18. I. R. Galatzer-Levy and R. A. Bryant, "636,120 Ways to Have Posttraumatic Stress Disorder," *Perspectives on Psychological Science* 8, no. 6 (2013): 651–662, https://doi.org/10.1177/1745691613504115.

19. R. J. McNally, "Progress and Controversy in the Study of Posttraumatic Stress Disorder," *Annual Review of Psychology* 54 (2003): 229–252.

20. McNally, "Progress and Controversy."

21. G. M. Rosen, "Traumatic Events, Criterion Creep, and the Creation of Pretraumatic Stress Disorder," *Scientific Review of Mental Health Practice* 3, no. 2 (2004).

22. Conservative estimates typically use retrospective reports and restricted definitions of trauma to include only the most obvious events. See N. Breslau, H. D. Chilcoat, R. C. Kessler, and G. C. Davis, "Previous Exposure to Trauma and PTSD Effects of Subsequent Trauma: Results from the Detroit Area Survey of Trauma," *American Journal of Psychiatry* 156, no. 6 (1999): 902–907, https://doi.org/10.1176/ajp.156.6.902; F. H. Norris, "Epidemiology of Trauma: Frequency and Impact of Different Potentially Traumatic Events on Different Demographic Groups," *Journal of Consulting and Clinical Psychology* 60, no. 3 (1992): 409–418. A limitation of these studies is that people do forget traumas and also experience traumatic events not included in the study list. Studies using more sensitive measures, such as weekly assessments over many years, suggest that exposure to potentially traumatic events is much more frequent. See K. M. Lalande and G. A. Bonanno, "Retrospective Memory Bias for the Frequency of Potentially Traumatic Events: A Prospective Study," *Psychological Trauma-Theory Research Practice and Policy* 3, no. 2 (2011): 165–170, https://doi.org/10.1037/a0020847.

23. NBC's show *Trauma* aired in 2009–2010 (see www.nbc.com/trauma). The online video game *Trauma* was designed by Krystian Majewski (see www.traumagame.com).

24. For example, see *Psychology Today*'s page "Trauma," www.psychologytoday.com/basics/trauma.

25. David J. Morris, *The Evil Hours* (New York: Houghton Mifflin Harcourt, 2015), 2, 42.

Chapter 2: Finding Resilience

1. C. S. Holling, "Resilience and Stability of Ecological Systems," *Annual Review of Ecology and Systematics* (1973): 1–23.

2. N. Garmezy and K. Neuchterlein, "Invulnerable Children: The Fact and Fiction of Competence and Disadvantage," *American Journal of Orthopsychiatry* 42 (1972): 328; J. Kagan, "Resilience in Cognitive Development," *Ethos* 3, no. 2

(1975): 231–247; L. B. Murphy, "Coping, Vulnerability, and Resilience in Child-hood," in *Coping and Adaptation*, ed. G. V. Coelho, D. A. Hamburg, and J. E. Adams, 69–100 (New York: Basic Books, 1974); Emmy E. Werner, Jessie M. Bi-erman, and Fern E. French, *The Children of Kauai: A Longitudinal Study from the Prenatal Period to Age Ten* (Honolulu: University of Hawaii Press, 1971).

3. M. Rutter, "Protective Factors in Children's Responses to Stress and Disadvantage," in *Primary Prevention of Psychopathology*, vol. 3, *Social Competence in Children*, ed. M. W. Kent and J. E. Rolf, 49–74 (Lebanon, NH: University Press of New England, 1979); Emmy E. Werner and Ruth S. Smith, *Vulnerable but Invincible: A Study of Resilient Children* (New York: McGraw-Hill, 1982); E. E. Werner, "Risk, Resilience, and Recovery: Perspec-tives from the Kauai Longitudinal Study," *Development and Psychopathology* 5, no. 4 (1993): 503–515.

4. Herbert G. Birch and Joan Dye Gussow, *Disadvantaged Children: Health, Nutrition, and School Failure* (New York: Harcourt, Brace, and World, 1970); Children's Defense Fund, *Maternal and Child Health Date Book: The Health of America's Children* (Washington, DC: US Government Printing Office, 1986); N. Garmezy, "Resiliency and Vulnerability to Adverse Developmental Outcomes Associated with Poverty," *American Behavioral Scientist* 34 (1991): 416–430.

5. J. G. Noll, L. A. Horowitz, G. A. Bonanno, P. K. Trickett, and F. W. Put-nam, "Revictimization and Self-Harm in Females Who Experienced Childhood Sexual Abuse: Results from a Prospective Study," *Journal of Interpersonal Violence* 18, no. 12 (2003): 1452–1471; Judith Herman, *Trauma and Recovery* (New York: Basic Books, 1992).

6. A. S. Masten, K. M. Best, and N. Garmezy, "Resilience and Develop-ment: Contributions from the Study of Children Who Overcome Adversity," *Development and Psychopathology* 2, no. 4 (1990): 425–444; Werner, "Risk, Re-silience, and Recovery"; E. E. Werner, "Resilience in Development," *Current Di-rections in Psychological Science* 4, no. 3 (1995): 81–85; Suniya S. Luthar, ed., *Resilience and Vulnerability: Adaptation in the Context of Childhood Adversities* (New York: Cambridge University Press, 2003); M. Rutter, "Psychosocial Re-silience and Protective Mechanisms," *American Journal of Orthopsychiatry* 57, no. 3 (1987): 316–331; S. Fergus and M. A. Zimmerman, "Adolescent Resil-ience: A Framework for Understanding Healthy Development in the Face of Risk," *Annual Review of Public Health* 26, no. 1 (2004): 399–419, https://doi.org/10.1146/annurev.publhealth.26.021304.144357; A. DiRago and G. Vail-lant, "Resilience in Inner City Youth: Childhood Predictors of Occupational Sta-tus Across the Lifespan," *Journal of Youth and Adolescence* 36, no. 1 (2007): 61–70, https://doi.org/10.1007/s10964-006-9132-8.

7. A. M. Masten, "Ordinary Magic: Resilience Processes in Development," *American Psychologist* 56 (2001): 227–238. The term "superkids" was used in the title of a book review on resilience. See S. E. Buggie, "Superkids of the Ghetto," *Contemporary Psychology* 40 (1995): 1164–1165.

8. Ann S. Masten, *Ordinary Magic: Resilience in Development* (New York: Guilford Publications, 2014).

9. Masten, "Ordinary Magic."

10. Masten et al., "Resilience and Development," 434.

11. Masten et al., "Resilience and Development."

12. Masten et al., "Resilience and Development," 434; M. S. Burton, A. A. Cooper, N. C. Feeny, and L. A. Zoellner, "The Enhancement of Natural Resilience in Trauma Interventions," *Journal of Contemporary Psychotherapy* 45, no. 4 (2015): 193–204.

13. George A. Bonanno, *The Other Side of Sadness*, rev. ed. (New York: Basic Books, 2019).

14. C. B. Wortman and R. C. Silver, "The Myths of Coping with Loss," *Journal of Consulting and Clinical Psychology* 57, no. 3 (1989): 349–357.

15. See G. A. Bonanno, D. Keltner, A. Holen, and M. J. Horowitz, "When Avoiding Unpleasant Emotions Might Not Be Such a Bad Thing: Verbal-Autonomic Response Dissociation and Midlife Conjugal Bereavement," *Journal of Personality and Social Psychology* 69, no. 5 (1995): 975–989; G. A. Bonanno and D. Keltner, "Facial Expressions of Emotion and the Course of Conjugal Bereavement," *Journal of Abnormal Psychology* 106, no. 1 (1997): 126–137; D. Keltner and G. A. Bonanno, "A Study of Laughter and Dissociation: Distinct Correlates of Laughter and Smiling During Bereavement," *Journal of Personality and Social Psychology* 73, no. 4 (1997): 687–702; G. A. Bonanno, H. Znoj, H. I. Siddique, and M. J. Horowitz, "Verbal-Autonomic Dissociation and Adaptation to Midlife Conjugal Loss: A Follow-up at 25 Months," *Cognitive Therapy and Research* 23, no. 6 (1999): 605–624.

16. See Bonanno, *Other Side of Sadness*.

17. Erica Goode and Emily Eakin, "Threats and Responses: The Doctors; Mental Health: The Profession Tests Its Limits," *New York Times*, September 11, 2002.

18. Sarah Graham, "9/11: The Psychological Aftermath," *Scientific American*, November 12, 2001.

19. Goode and Eakin, "Threats and Responses."

20. Graham, "9/11."

21. M. A. Schuster, B. D. Stein, L. H. Jaycox, R. L. Collins, G. N. Marshall, M. N. Elliott, A. J. Zhou, D. E. Kanouse, J. L. Morrison, and S. H. Berry, "A National Survey of Stress Reactions After the September 11, 2001, Terrorist Attacks," *New England Journal of Medicine* 345, no. 20 (2001): 1507–1512, https://doi.org/10.1056/NEJM200111153452024.

22. S. Galea, H. Resnick, J. Ahern, J. Gold, M. Bucuvalas, D. Kilpatrick, J. Stuber, and D. Vlahov, "Posttraumatic Stress Disorder in Manhattan, New York City, After the September 11th Terrorist Attacks," *Journal of Urban Health* 79, no. 3 (2002): 340–353.

23. S. Galea, J. Ahern, H. Resnick, D. Kilpatrick, M. Bucuvalas, J. Gold, and D. Vlahov, "Psychological Sequelae of the September 11 Terrorist Attacks in New York City," *New England Journal of Medicine* 346, no. 13 (2002): 982–987.

24. S. Galea, D. Vlahov, H. Resnick, J. Ahern, E. Susser, J. Gold, M. Bucu-valas, and D. Kilpatrick, "Trends of Probable Post-Traumatic Stress Disorder in New York City After the September 11 Terrorist Attacks," *American Journal of Epidemiology* 158, no. 6 (2003): 514–524.

25. Galea et al., "Trends of Probable Post-Traumatic Stress Disorder in New York City."

26. Goode and Eakin, "Threats and Responses."

27. Goode and Eakin, "Threats and Responses."

28. "Mycosis Fungoides: A Rash That Can Be Cancer," Stanford Health Care, March 24, 2014, https://stanfordhealthcare.org/newsroom/articles/2014/mycosis-fungoides.html.

29. H. S. Resnick, D. G. Kilpatrick, B. S. Dansky, B. E. Saunders, and C. L. Best, "Prevalence of Civilian Trauma and Posttraumatic Stress Disorder in a Representative National Sample of Women," *Journal of Consulting and Clinical Psychology* 61, no. 6 (1993): 984–991, https://doi.org/10.1037/0022-006X.61 .6.984; C. Blanco, "Epidemiology of PTSD," in *Post-Traumatic Stress Disorder*, ed. D. J. Stein, M. Friedman, and C. Blanco, 49–74 (West Sussex, UK: Wiley Online Library, 2011); R. C. Kessler, A. Sonnega, E. Bromet, M. Hughes, and C. B. Nelson, "Posttraumatic Stress Disorder in the National Comorbidity Survey," *Archives of General Psychiatry* 52, no. 12 (1995): 1048–1060.

30. Patricia Resick, in Jennifer Daw, "What Have We Learned Since 9/11? Psychologists Share Their Thoughts on Lessons Learned and Where to Go from Here," *Monitor on Psychology* 33, no. 8 (September 2002), www.apa.org/monitor /sep02/learned.

31. Many trauma experts believe that extreme traumatic stress in the first weeks after a potentially traumatic event is a clinical condition that leads to PTSD. The strength of this belief eventually led to the creation of a separate diagnostic category, acute stress disorder (ASD), for the express purpose of identifying and treating early severe traumatic stress reactions. However, the research on ASD failed to support its predictive relationship to later PTSD. Only about 20 percent of people exposed to a potentially traumatic event meet the criteria for ASD, and most of those people do not develop PTSD. In other words, ASD does not reliably identify who will and who will not eventually develop PTSD. Some evidence suggests that ASD may still prove useful by identifying individuals with extreme levels of traumatic stress who might benefit from some form of early treatment. However, this research has focused exclusively on treatment-seeking individuals and has not evaluated the possibility that, since most people meeting criteria for ASD recover spontaneously, some individuals might be harmed by an unnecessary clinical intervention. For more on ASD, see R. A. Bryant, "The Current Evidence for Acute Stress Disorder," *Current Psychiatry Reports* 20, no. 12 (2018): 111. For more on possible harmful effects of psychological treatments, see S. O. Lilienfeld, "Psychological Treatments That Cause Harm," *Perspectives on Psychological Science* 2, no. 1 (2007): 53–70.

32. Elizabeth F. Howell, *The Dissociative Mind* (New York: Routledge, 2013), 4.

33. Jasmin Lee Cori, *Healing from Trauma: A Survivor's Guide to Understanding Your Symptoms and Reclaiming Your Life* (New York: Da Capo, 2008).

34. Mark Epstein, *The Trauma of Everyday Life* (New York: Penguin, 2013), 1.

35. J. Shedler, M. Mayman, and M. Manis, "The Illusion of Mental Health," *American Psychologist* 48, no. 11 (1993): 1117–1131.

36. A. Tversky and D. Kahneman, "Judgment Under Uncertainty: Heuristics and Biases," *Science* 185, no. 4157 (1974): 1124–1131, https://doi.org/10.1126/science.185.4157.1124.

37. Amos Tversky and Daniel Kahneman, "Evidential Impact of Base Rates," in *Judgment Under Uncertainty: Heuristics and Biases*, ed. Daniel Kahneman, Paul Slovic, and Amos Tversky, 153–163 (Cambridge: Cambridge University Press, 1982).

38. Tversky and Kahneman, "Evidential Impact of Base Rates"; Derek J. Koehler, Lyle Brenner, and Dale Griffin, "The Calibration of Expert Judgment: Heuristics and Biases Beyond the Laboratory," in *Heuristics and Biases: The Psychology of Intuitive Judgment*, ed. Thomas Gilovich, Dale W. Griffin, and Daniel Kahneman, 686–715 (Cambridge: Cambridge University Press, 2002); S. Ægisdóttir, M. J. White, P. M. Spengler, A. S. Maugherman, L. A. Anderson, R. S. Cook, C. N. Nichols, et al., "The Meta-Analysis of Clinical Judgment Project: Fifty-Six Years of Accumulated Research on Clinical Versus Statistical Prediction," *Counseling Psychologist* 34, no. 3 (2006): 341–382; J. Z. Ayanian and D. M. Berwick, "Do Physicians Have a Bias Toward Action? A Classic Study Revisited," *Medical Decision Making* 11, no. 3 (1991): 154–158, https://doi.org/10.1177/0272989X9101100302; P. Msaouel, T. Kappos, A. Tasoulis, A. P. Apostolopoulos, I. Lekkas, E.-S. Tripodaki, and N. C. Keramaris, "Assessment of Cognitive Biases and Biostatistics Knowledge of Medical Residents: A Multicenter, Cross-Sectional Questionnaire Study," *Medical Education Online* 19 (2014), https://doi.org/10.3402/meo.v19.23646; A. S. Elstein, "Heuristics and Biases: Selected Errors in Clinical Reasoning," *Academic Medicine* 74, no. 7 (1999); H. N. Garb, "The Representativeness and Past-Behavior Heuristics in Clinical Judgment," *Professional Psychology: Research and Practice* 27, no. 3 (1996): 272–277, https://doi.org/10.1037/0735-7028.27.3.272.

39. Garb, "Representativeness and Past-Behavior Heuristics."

40. K. Hek, A. Demirkan, J. Lahti, A. Terracciano, A. Teumer, M. C. Cornelis, N. Amin, et al., "A Genome-Wide Association Study of Depressive Symptoms," *Biological Psychiatry* 73, no. 7 (2013): 667–678, https://doi.org/10.1016/j.biopsych.2012.09.033; S. Tomitaka, Y. Kawasaki, K. Ide, H. Yamada, H. Miyake, and T. A. Furukawa, "Distribution of Total Depressive Symptoms Scores and Each Depressive Symptom Item in a Sample of Japanese Employees," *PLoS ONE* 11, no. 1 (2016): e0147577–e0147577, https://doi.org/10.1371/journal.pone.0147577.

41. G. A. Bonanno, "Loss, Trauma, and Human Resilience: Have We Underestimated the Human Capacity to Thrive After Extremely Aversive Events?" *American Psychologist* 59, no. (2004): 20–28.

42. I. R. Galatzer-Levy, S. A. Huang, and G. A. Bonanno, "Trajectories of Resilience and Dysfunction Following Potential Trauma: A Review and Statistical Evaluation," *Clinical Psychology Review* 63 (2018): 41–55.

43. Naval Health Research Center, "The Largest DoD Population-Based Military Health Study Launched Next Survey Cycle, Hopes to Enroll Military Members and Spouses," press release, July 19, 2011.

44. See G. A. Bonanno, A. D. Mancini, J. L. Horton, T. Powell, C. A. Leard-Mann, E. J. Boyko, T. S. Wells, T. I. Hooper, G. Gackstetter, and T. C. Smith, "Trajectories of Trauma Symptoms and Resilience in Deployed U.S. Military Service Members: A Prospective Cohort Study," *British Journal of Psychiatry* 200 (2012): 317–323. See also C. J. Donoho, G. A. Bonanno, B. Porter, L. Kearney, and T. M. Powell, "A Decade of War: Prospective Trajectories of Posttraumatic Stress Disorder Symptoms Among Deployed US Military Personnel and the Influence of Combat Exposure," *American Journal of Epidemiology* 186, no. 12 (2017): 1310–1318, https://doi.org/10.1093/aje/kwx318.

45. T. A. DeRoon-Cassini, A. D. Mancini, M. D. Rusch, and G. A. Bonanno, "Psychopathology and Resilience Following Traumatic Injury: A Latent Growth Mixture Model Analysis," *Rehabilitation Psychology* 55, no. 1 (2010): 1–11, https://doi.org/10.1037/a0018601; R. A. Bryant, A. Nickerson, M. Creamer, M. O'Donnell, D. Forbes, I. Galatzer-Levy, A. C. McFarlane, and D. Silove, "Trajectory of Post-Traumatic Stress Following Traumatic Injury: 6-Year Follow-up," *British Journal of Psychiatry* 206, no. 5 (2015): 417–423, https://doi.org/10.1192/bjp.bp.114.145516; G. A. Bonanno, P. Kennedy, I. R. Galatzer-Levy, P. Lude, and M. L. Elfström, "Trajectories of Resilience, Depression, and Anxiety Following Spinal Cord Injury," *Rehabilitation Psychology* 57, no. 3 (2012): 236–247, https://doi.org/10.1037/a0029256.

46. For cancer trajectories, see C. L. Burton, I. R. Galatzer-Levy, and G. A. Bonanno, "Treatment Type and Demographic Characteristics as Predictors for Cancer Adjustment: Prospective Trajectories of Depressive Symptoms in a Population Sample," *Health Psychology* 34 (2015): 602–609, https://doi.org/10.1037/hea0000145; W. W. T. Lam, G. A. Bonanno, A. D. Mancini, S. Ho, M. Chan, W. K. Hung, A. Or, and R. Fielding, "Trajectories of Psychological Distress Among Chinese Women Diagnosed with Breast Cancer," *Psycho-Oncology* 19, no. 10 (2010): 1044–1051, https://doi.org/10.1002/pon.1658. For heart attack trajectories, see I. R. Galatzer-Levy and G. A. Bonanno, "Optimism and Death: Predicting the Course and Consequences of Depression Trajectories in Response to Heart Attack," *Psychological Science* 24, no. 12 (2014): 2177–2188, https://doi.org/10.1177/0956797614551750; L. Meli, J. L. Birk, D. Edmondson, and G. A. Bonanno, "Trajectories of Posttraumatic Stress Symptoms in Patients with Confirmed and Rule-Out Acute Coronary Syndrome," *General Hospital Psychiatry* 62 (2019).

47. For recent bereavement studies, see F. Maccallum, I. R. Galatzer-Levy, and G. A. Bonanno, "Trajectories of Depression Following Spousal and Child Bereavement: A Comparison of the Heterogeneity in Outcomes," *Journal of Psychiatric Research* 69 (2015): 72–79, https://doi.org/10.1016/j.jpsychires.2015.07.017; G. A. Bonanno and M. Malgaroli, "Trajectories of Grief: Comparing Symptoms from the DSM-5 and ICD-11 Diagnoses," *Depression and Anxiety* 37, no. 1 (2020): 17–25. For recent studies of divorce and unemployment, see M. Malgaroli, I. R. Galatzer-Levy, and G. A. Bonanno, "Heterogeneity in Trajectories of Depression in Response to Divorce Is Associated with Differential Risk for Mortality," *Clinical Psychological Science* 5, no. 5 (2017): 843–850, https://doi.org/10.1177/2167702617705951; C. A. Stolove, I. R. Galatzer-Levy, and G. A. Bonanno, "Emergence of Depression Following Job Loss Prospectively Predicts Lower Rates of Reemployment," *Psychiatry Research* 253 (2017): 79–83.

Chapter 3: More Than Meets the Eye

1. I. R. Galatzer-Levy, S. H. Huang, and G. A. Bonanno, "Trajectories of Resilience and Dysfunction Following Potential Trauma: A Review and Statistical Evaluation," *Clinical Psychology Review* 63 (2018): 41–55, https://doi.org/10.1016/j.cpr.2018.05.008.

2. F. H. Norris, M. J. Friedman, and P. J. Watson, "60,000 Disaster Victims Speak. Part II: Summary and Implications of the Disaster Mental Health Research," *Psychiatry-Interpersonal and Biological Processes* 65, no. 3 (2002): 240–260, https://doi.org/10.1521/psyc.65.3.240.20169.

3. G. A. Bonanno, S. Galea, A. Bucciarelli, and D. Vlahov, "Psychological Resilience After Disaster: New York City in the Aftermath of the September 11th Terrorist Attack," *Psychological Science* 17, no. 3 (2006): 181–186, https://doi.org/10.1111/j.1467-9280.2006.01682.x.

4. C. J. Donoho, G. A. Bonanno, B. Porter, L. Kearney, and T. M. Powell, "A Decade of War: Prospective Trajectories of Posttraumatic Stress Disorder Symptoms Among Deployed US Military Personnel and the Influence of Combat Exposure," *American Journal of Epidemiology* 186, no. 12 (2017): 1310–1318, https://doi.org/10.1093/aje/kwx318.

5. For reviews of effect sizes in trauma severity on trauma outcomes, see C. R. Brewin, B. Andrews, and J. D. Valentine, "Meta-Analysis of Risk Factors for Posttraumatic Stress Disorder in Trauma-Exposed Adults," *Journal of Consulting and Clinical Psychology* 68, no. 5 (2000): 748–766; E. J. Ozer, S. R. Best, T. L. Lipsey, and D. S. Weiss, "Predictors of Posttraumatic Stress Disorder and Symptoms in Adults: A Meta-Analysis," *Psychological Bulletin* 129, no. 1 (2003): 52–73. For an example of a study showing that trauma is modified by other factors, see E. Levy-Gigi, G. A. Bonanno, A. R. Shapiro, G. Richter-Levin, S. Kéri, and G. Sheppes, "Emotion Regulatory Flexibility Sheds Light on the Elusive Relationship Between Repeated Traumatic Exposure and Posttraumatic Stress Disorder

Symptoms," *Clinical Psychological Science* 4, no. 1 (2015): 28–39. For examples of studies reporting no influence of trauma severity, see A. Boals, Z. Trost, E. Rainey, M. L. Foreman, and A. M. Warren, "Severity of Traumatic Injuries Predicting Psychological Outcomes: A Surprising Lack of Empirical Evidence," *Journal of Anxiety Disorders* 50, (2017): 1–6, https://doi.org/10.1016/j.janxdis.2017.04.004; Y. Neria, A. Besser, D. Kiper, and M. Westphal, "A Longitudinal Study of Posttraumatic Stress Disorder, Depression, and Generalized Anxiety Disorder in Israeli Civilians Exposed to War Trauma," *Journal of Traumatic Stress* 23, no. 3 (2010): 322–330.

Chapter 4: The Resilience Paradox

1. Predictors of resilience touted in popular books, on websites, and in the media were gleaned from the following: Sheryl Sandberg and Adam Grant, *Option B: Facing Adversity, Building Resilience, and Finding Joy* (New York: Knopf, 2017); Zelana Montminy, *21 Days to Resilience: How to Transcend the Daily Grind, Deal with the Tough Stuff, and Discover Your Inner Strength* (New York: HarperOne, 2016); Elaine Miller-Karas, *Building Resilience to Trauma: The Trauma and Community Resiliency Models* (New York: Routledge, 2015); Steven M. Southwick and Dennis S. Charney, *Resilience: The Science of Mastering Life's Greatest Challenges* (Cambridge: Cambridge University Press, 2012); Glenn R. Schiraldi, *The Resilience Workbook: Essential Skills to Recover from Stress, Trauma, and Adversity* (Oakland, CA: New Harbinger, 2017); Donald Robertson, *Build Your Resilience: CBT, Mindfulness and Stress Management to Survive and Thrive in Any Situation* (London: Hodder Education, 2012); Kelly Ann McNight, *The Resilience Way: Overcome the Unexpected and Build an Extraordinary Life . . . on Your Own Terms!* (independently published, 2019). Websites and magazine articles included the following: Romeo Vitelli, "What Makes Us Resilient?," *Psychology Today*, April 10, 2018, www.psychologytoday.com/us/blog/media-spotlight/201804/what-makes-us-resilient; Kendra Cherry, "Characteristics of Resilient People," *Very Well Mind*, April 28, 2020, www.verywellmind.com/characteristics-of-resilience-2795062; Brad Waters, "10 Traits of Emotionally Resilient People," *Psychology Today*, May 21, 2013, www.psychologytoday.com/us/blog/design-your-path/201305/10-traits-emotionally-resilient-people; Kendra Cherry, "10 Ways to Build Your Resilience," *Very Well Mind*, January 24, 2020, www.verywellmind.com/ways-to-become-more-resilient-2795063; Leslie Riopel, "Resilient Skills, Factors and Strategies of the Resilient Person," *Positive Psychology*, September 19, 2020, https://positivepsychology.com/resilience-skills; "What Makes Some People More Resilient Than Others," *Exploring Your Mind*, June 5, 2016, https://exploringyourmind.com/makes-people-resilient-others; Allan Schwartz, "Are You Emotionally Resilient?," *Mental Help* (blog), October 12, 2019, www.mentalhelp.net/blogs/are-you-emotionally-resilient; LaRae Quy, "4 Powerful Ways You Can Make Yourself More Resilient—Now," *The Ladders*, January 11, 2019,

www.theladders.com/career-advice/4-powerful-ways-you-can-make-yourself -more-resilient-now; "5 Steps to a More Resilient You," *Psych Central,* January 30, 2011, https://psychcentral.com/blog/5-steps-to-a-more-resilient-you#1; "Being Resilient," *Your Life Your Voice,* October 16, 2019, www.yourlifeyourvoice.org /Pages/tip-being-resilient.aspx.

2. J. F. P. Peres, A. Moreira-Almeida, A. G. Nasello, and H. G. Koenig, "Spirituality and Resilience in Trauma Victims," *Journal of Religion and Health* 46, no. 3 (2007): 343–350 (quote from 343), https://doi.org/10.1007/s10943-006-9103-0.

3. Olivia Goldhill, "Psychologists Have Found That a Spiritual Outlook Makes Humans More Resilient," *Quartz,* January 30, 2016, https://qz.com/606564 /psychologists-have-found-that-a-spiritual-outlook-makes-humans-universally -more-resilient-to-trauma.

4. For more on this topic, see H. R. Moody, "Is Religion Good for Your Health?," *Gerontologist* 46, no. 1 (2006): 147–149; J. T. Moore and M. M. Leach, "Dogmatism and Mental Health: A Comparison of the Religious and Secular," *Psychology of Religion and Spirituality* 8, no. 1 (2016): 54.

5. See J. H. Wortmann, C. L. Park, and D. Edmondson, "Trauma and PTSD Symptoms: Does Spiritual Struggle Mediate the Link?," *Psychological Trauma: Theory, Research, Practice and Policy* 3, no. 4 (2011): 442–452, https://doi.org /10.1037/a0021413; N. Caluori, J. C. Jackson, K. Gray, and M. Gelfand, "Conflict Changes How People View God," *Psychological Science* 31, no. 3 (2020): 280–292, https://doi.org/10.1177/0956797619895286.

6. R. W. Thompson, D. B. Arnkoff, and C. R. Glass, "Conceptualizing Mindfulness and Acceptance as Components of Psychological Resilience to Trauma," *Trauma, Violence, and Abuse* 12, no. 4 (2011): 220–235.

7. R. A. Baer, G. T. Smith, J. Hopkins, J. Krietemeyer, and L. Toney, "Using Self-Report Assessment Methods to Explore Facets of Mindfulness," *Assessment* 13, no. 1 (2006): 27–45.

8. On the general health benefits of mindfulness, see R. J. Davidson, J. Kabat-Zinn, J. Schumacher, M. Rosenkranz, D. Muller, S. F. Santorelli, F. Urbanowski, A. Harrington, K. Bonus, and J. F. Sheridan, "Alterations in Brain and Immune Function Produced by Mindfulness Meditation," *Psychosomatic Medicine* 65, no. 4 (2003). See also K. W. Brown, R. M. Ryan, and J. D. Creswell, "Mindfulness: Theoretical Foundations and Evidence for Its Salutary Effects," *Psychological Inquiry* 18, no. 4 (2007): 211–237; J. D. Creswell, "Mindfulness Interventions," *Annual Review of Psychology* 68 (2017): 491–516; J. Suttie, "Five Ways Mindfulness Meditation Is Good for Your Health," *Greater Good Magazine,* October 2018, https://greatergood.berkeley.edu/article/item/five_ways_mindfulness _meditation_is_good_for_your_health.

9. On the benefits of mindfulness in clinical intervention, see J. D. Teasdale, Z. V. Segal, J. M. G. Williams, V. A. Ridgeway, J. M. Soulsby, and M. A. Lau, "Prevention of Relapse/Recurrence in Major Depression by Mindfulness-Based Cognitive Therapy," *Journal of Consulting and Clinical Psychology* 68, no. 4 (2000): 615; S. G. Hofmann, A. T. Sawyer, A. A. Witt, and D. Oh, "The Effect

of Mindfulness-Based Therapy on Anxiety and Depression: A Meta-Analytic Review," *Journal of Consulting and Clinical Psychology* 78, no. 2 (2010): 169–183, https://doi.org/10.1037/a0018555; B. Khoury, T. Lecomte, G. Fortin, M. Masse, P. Therien, V. Bouchard, M.-A. Chapleau, K. Paquin, and S. G. Hofmann, "Mindfulness-Based Therapy: A Comprehensive Meta-Analysis," *Clinical Psychology Review* 33, no. 6 (2013): 763–771; J. D. Creswell, "Mindfulness Interventions," *Annual Review of Psychology* 68 (2017): 491–516.

10. R. W. Thompson, D. B. Arnkoff, and C. R. Glass, "Conceptualizing Mindfulness and Acceptance as Components of Psychological Resilience to Trauma," *Trauma, Violence, and Abuse* 12, no. 4 (2011): 220–235.

11. Quote from the abstract of N. T. Van Dam, M. K. van Vugt, D. R. Vago, L. Schmalzl, C. D. Saron, A. Olendzki, T. Meissner, et al., "Mind the Hype: A Critical Evaluation and Prescriptive Agenda for Research on Mindfulness and Meditation," *Perspectives on Psychological Science* 13, no. 1 (2018): 36–61. On the possible side-effects of mindfulness meditation, see M. K. Lustyk, N. Chawla, R. Nolan, and G. Marlatt, "Mindfulness Meditation Research: Issues of Participant Screening, Safety Procedures, and Researcher Training," *Advances in Mind-Body Medicine* 24, no. 1 (2009): 20–30.

12. We will spend more time on these factors later in the book. For more information and research evidence on these predictors, see G. A. Bonanno, M. Westphal, and A. D. Mancini, "Resilience to Loss and Potential Trauma," *Annual Review of Clinical Psychology* 7 (2011), https://doi.org/10.1146/annurev -clinpsy-032210-104526; G. A. Bonanno, C. R. Brewin, K. Kaniasty, and A. M. La Greca, "Weighing the Costs of Disaster: Consequences, Risks, and Resilience in Individuals, Families, and Communities," *Psychological Science in the Public Interest* 11, no. 1 (2010): 1–49; G. A. Bonanno, S. A. Romero, and S. I. Klein, "The Temporal Elements of Psychological Resilience: An Integrative Framework for the Study of Individuals, Families, and Communities," *Psychological Inquiry* 26, no. 2 (2015): 139–169, https://doi.org/10.1080/1047840X.2015.992677. For evidence for genetic profiles that differentiate resilience and the other trajectories, see K. Schultebraucks, K. W. Choi, I. G. Galatzer-Levy, and G. A. Bonanno, "Discriminating Heterogeneous Trajectories of Resilience and Depression After Major Stressors Using Polygenic Scores: A Deep Learning Approach," *JAMA Psychiatry* (in press).

13. I've simplified the idea of effect sizes for the sake of clarity in this discussion. The idea is somewhat more complex than I have suggested. It's not always easy to determine effect sizes in some types of statistical analyses, for example, in which case we can only calculate proxy effect sizes. Also, it's worth noting that effect sizes seem larger when only one or two predictors are examined. That's because other related factors that might also predict resilience had not been considered. When we are able to examine many possible predictors in the same analysis, as in a so-called multivariate analysis, we can increase the overall variance explained. In other words, we can somewhat better explain who will be resilient

and who not. However, because many predictors tend to correlate to some extent with each other, the portion explained by any one predictor typically gets smaller.

14. For a discussion of these predictors and the quality of evidence behind them, see, again, Bonanno et al., "Resilience to Loss and Potential Trauma"; Bonanno et al., "Weighing the Costs of Disaster"; and Bonanno et al., "The Temporal Elements of Psychological Resilience."

15. W. Mischel and Y. Shoda, "A Cognitive-Affective System Theory of Personality: Reconceptualizing Situations, Dispositions, Dynamics, and Invariance in Personality Structure," *Psychological Review* 102, no. 2 (1995): 246–268, https://doi.org/10.1037/0033-295X.102.2.246; W. Mischel, "Toward a Cognitive Social Learning Reconceptualization of Personality," *Psychological Review* 80, no. 4 (1973): 252–283, https://doi.org/10.1037/h0035002; W. Mischel, Y. Shoda, and R. Mendoza-Denton, "Situation-Behavior Profiles as a Locus of Consistency in Personality," *Current Directions in Psychological Science* 11, no. 2 (2002): 50–54; W. Mischel, *The Marshmallow Test: Why Self-Control Is the Engine of Success* (New York: Little, Brown, 2014).

16. For further discussion of cost-benefit analyses in nature, see T. Kalisky, E. Dekel, and U. Alon, "Cost-Benefit Theory and Optimal Design of Gene Regulation Functions," *Physical Biology* 4, no. 4 (2007): 229; H. A. Orr, "The Genetic Theory of Adaptation: A Brief History," *Nature Reviews Genetics* 6, no. 2 (2005): 119–127, https://doi.org/10.1038/nrg1523; J. S. Brown and T. L. Vincent, "Evolution of Cooperation with Shared Costs and Benefits," *Proceedings of the Royal Society B: Biological Sciences* 275, no. 1646 (2008): 1985–1994; A. V. Georgiev, A. C. E. Klimczuk, D. M. Traficonte, and D. Maestripieri, "When Violence Pays: A Cost-Benefit Analysis of Aggressive Behavior in Animals and Humans," *Evolutionary Psychology* 11, no. 3 (2013): 678–699.

17. Charles Darwin, *On the Origin of Species, by Means of Natural Selection* (London: John Murray, 1859).

18. Letter from Darwin to botanist Asa Gray, April 3, 1860, The Darwin Correspondence Project, University of Cambridge, www.darwinproject.ac.uk/letter/DCP-LETT-2743.xml.

19. Charles Darwin, *The Descent of Man, and Selection in Relation to Sex* (London: John Murray, 1871).

20. Darwin, *Descent of Man*, 141.

21. Richard O. Prum, *The Evolution of Beauty: How Darwin's Forgotten Theory of Mate Choice Shapes the Animal World* (New York: Penguin Random House, 2017); M. Petrie and T. Halliday, "Experimental and Natural Changes in the Peacock's (*Pavo cristatus*) Train Can Affect Mating Success," *Behavioral Ecology and Sociobiology* 35, no. 3 (1994): 213–217, https://doi.org/10.1007/BF00167962.

22. Although it was long believed that cheetahs stop running because they overheat, more recent research suggests they have something akin to a severe stress response. For more on cheetahs, see R. S. Hetem, D. Mitchell, B. A. de Witt, L. G. Fick, L. C. R. Meyer, S. K. Maloney, and A. Fuller, "Cheetah Do Not

Abandon Hunts Because They Overheat," *Biology Letters* 9, no. 5 (2013): 20130472, https://doi.org/10.1098/rsbl.2013.0472; T. Y. Hubel, J. P. Myatt, N. R. Jordan, O. P. Dewhirst, J. W. McNutt, and A. M. Wilson, "Energy Cost and Return for Hunting in African Wild Dogs and Cheetahs," *Nature Communications* 7, no. 1 (2016): 11034, https://doi.org/10.1038/ncomms11034; R. Nuwer, "Cheetahs Spend 90 Percent of Their Days Sitting Around," *Smithsonian*, October 2014; "Adaptations to Speed," Dell Cheetah Center, Zambia, www.dccafrica .co.za/cheetah-facts/adaptations-to-speed.

23. On the good-bad taxonomy in coping and emotion regulation, see A. Aldao and S. Nolen-Hoeksema, "When Are Adaptive Strategies Most Predictive of Psychopathology?," *Journal of Abnormal Psychology* 121, no. 1 (2012): 276–281, https://doi.org/10.1037/a0023598; C. A. Smith, K. A. Wallston, K. A. Dwyer, and W. Dowdy, "Beyond Good and Bad Coping: A Multidimensional Examination of Coping with Pain in Persons with Rheumatoid Arthritis," *Annals of Behavioral Medicine* 19, no. 1 (1997): 11–21.

24. For a more detailed account of this research, see J. E. Schwartz, J. Neale, C. Marco, S. S. Shiffman, and A. A. Stone, "Does Trait Coping Exist? A Momentary Assessment Approach to the Evaluation of Traits," *Journal of Personality and Social Psychology* 77, no. 2 (1999): 360–369, https://doi.org/10.1037/0022 -3514.77.2.360; A. A. Stone, J. E. Schwartz, J. M. Neale, S. Shiffman, C. A. Marco, M. Hickcox, J. Paty, L. S. Porter, and L. J. Cruise, "A Comparison of Coping Assessed by Ecological Momentary Assessment and Retrospective Recall," *Journal of Personality and Social Psychology* 74, no. 6 (1998): 1670.

25. For more on these findings, see J. L. Austenfeld and A. L. Stanton, "Coping Through Emotional Approach: A New Look at Emotion, Coping, and Health-Related Outcomes," *Journal of Personality* 72, no. 6 (2004): 1335–1364, https://doi.org/10.1111/j.1467-6494.2004.00299; J. Smyth and S. J. Lepore, *The Writing Cure: How Expressive Writing Promotes Health and Emotional Well-Being* (Washington, DC: American Psychological Association, 2002); B. E. Compas, C. J. Forsythe, and B. M. Wagner, "Consistency and Variability in Causal Attributions and Coping with Stress," *Cognitive Therapy and Research* 12, no. 3 (1988): 305–320, https://doi.org/10.1007/bf01176192; D. G. Kaloupek, H. White, and M. Wong, "Multiple Assessment of Coping Strategies Used by Volunteer Blood Donors: Implications for Preparatory Training," *Journal of Behavioral Medicine* 7, no. 1 (1984): 35–60, https://doi.org/10.1007/BF00845346.

26. T. L. Webb, E. Miles, and P. Sheeran, "Dealing with Feeling: A Meta-Analysis of the Effectiveness of Strategies Derived from the Process Model of Emotion Regulation," *Psychological Bulletin* 138, no. 4 (2012): 775–808, https:// doi.org/10.1037/a0027600.

27. G. Hein, G. Silani, K. Preuschoff, C. D. Batson, and T. Singer, "Neural Responses to Ingroup and Outgroup Members' Suffering Predict Individual Differences in Costly Helping," *Neuron* 68, no. 1 (2010): 149–160, https://doi .org/10.1016/j.neuron.2010.09.003; James C. Coyne, Camille B. Wortman, and Darrin R. Lehman, "The Other Side of Support: Emotional Overinvolvement

and Miscarried Helping," in *Marshaling Social Support: Formats, Processes, and Effects*, ed. Benjamin H. Gottlieb, 305–330 (Thousand Oaks, CA: Sage, 1988); J. C. Coyne, "Depression and the Response of Others," *Journal of Abnormal Psychology* 85 (1976): 186–193, https://doi.org/10.1037/0021-843X.85.2.186; E. D. Diminich and G. A. Bonanno, "Faces, Feelings, Words: Divergence Across Channels of Emotional Responding in Complicated Grief," *Journal of Abnormal Psychology* 123 (2014): 350–361.

28. A. S. Troy, A. J. Shallcross, and I. B. Mauss, "A Person-by-Situation Approach to Emotion Regulation: Cognitive Reappraisal Can Either Help or Hurt, Depending on the Context," *Psychological Science* 24, no. 2 (2013): 2505–2514, https://doi.org/10.1177/0956797613496434; G. Sheppes, S. Scheibe, G. Suri, P. Radu, J. Blechert, and J. J. Gross, "Emotion Regulation Choice: A Conceptual Framework and Supporting Evidence," *Journal of Experimental Psychology: General* 143, no. 1 (2014): 163–181, https://doi.org/10.1037/a0030831.

29. On coping research and theory, see R. S. Lazarus and S. Folkman, *Stress, Appraisal, and Coping* (New York: Springer, 1984); S. Folkman and J. T. Moskowitz, "Coping: Pitfalls and Promise," *Annual Review of Psychology* 55, no. 1 (2004): 745–774; C. S. Carver and J. Connor-Smith, "Personality and Coping," *Annual Review of Psychology* 61, no. 1 (2009): 679–704; C. Cheng, "Assessing Coping Flexibility in Real-Life and Laboratory Settings: A Multimethod Approach," *Journal of Personality and Social Psychology* 80, no. 5 (2001): 814–833. For emotion regulation, see J. J. Gross, "The Emerging Field of Emotion Regulation: An Integrative Review," *Review of General Psychology* 2, no. 3 (1998): 271–299; J. J. Gross, "Emotion Regulation: Past, Present, Future," *Cognition and Emotion* 13, no. 5 (1999): 551–573; A. Aldao, G. Sheppes, and J. J. Gross, "Emotion Regulation Flexibility," *Cognitive Therapy and Research* 39, no. 3 (2015): 263–278. For an integrative review of both coping and emotion regulation, see G. A. Bonanno and C. L. Burton, "Regulatory Flexibility: An Individual Differences Perspective on Coping and Emotion Regulation," *Perspectives on Psychological Science* 8, no. 6 (2013): 591–612, https://doi.org/10.1177/1745691613504116.

30. See G. A. Bonanno, "Resilience in the Face of Loss and Potential Trauma," *Current Directions in Psychological Science* 14, no. 3 (2005): 135–138; G. A. Bonanno, *The Other Side of Sadness: What the New Science of Bereavement Tells Us About Life After Loss* (New York: Basic Books, 2009).

31. Much of this impetus has sprung from the excellent research of Barbara Fredrickson. See, for example, Barbara L. Fredrickson and Laura E. Kurtz, "Cultivating Positive Emotions to Enhance Human Flourishing," in *Applied Positive Psychology: Improving Everyday Life, Health, Schools, Work, and Society*, ed. Stewart I. Donaldson, Mihaly Csikszentmihalyi, and Jeanne Nakamura, 35–47 (New York: Taylor and Francis, 2011); B. L. Fredrickson, "Cultivating Positive Emotions to Optimize Health and Well-Being," *Prevention and Treatment* 3, no. 1 (2000): 1a. But see also popular websites, such as Tony Robbins's blog, Mind and Meaning, where Robbins describes positive emotions and the "emotional seeds to plant in your garden to bring fulfillment and abundance to your life." Quoted

from Team Tony, "Cultivating Positive Emotions: 10 Emotional Seeds to Plant in Your Garden Now," Tony Robbins, www.tonyrobbins.com/mind-meaning /cultivating-positive-emotions.

32. For an excellent review of this literature, see J. Gruber, I. B. Mauss, and M. Tamir, "A Dark Side of Happiness? How, When, and Why Happiness Is Not Always Good," *Perspectives on Psychological Science* 6, no. 3 (2011): 222–233, https://doi.org/10.1177/1745691611406927. See also M. A. Davis, "Understanding the Relationship Between Mood and Creativity: A Meta-Analysis," *Organizational Behavior and Human Decision Processes* 108, no. 1 (2009): 25–38; M. Tamir, C. Mitchell, and J. J. Gross, "Hedonic and Instrumental Motives in Anger Regulation," *Psychological Science* 19, no. 4 (2008): 324–328, https://doi .org/10.1111/j.1467-9280.2008.02088.x; E. Diener, C. R. Colvin, W. G. Pavot, and A. Allman, "The Psychic Costs of Intense Positive Affect," *Journal of Personality and Social Psychology* 61, no. 3 (1991): 492; E. K. Kalokerinos, K. H. Greenaway, D. J. Pedder, and E. A. Margetts, "Don't Grin When You Win: The Social Costs of Positive Emotion Expression in Performance Situations," *Emotion* 14, no. 1 (2014): 180.

33. See A. Papa and G. A. Bonanno, "Smiling in the Face of Adversity: The Interpersonal and Intrapersonal Functions of Smiling," *Emotion* 8, no. 1 (2008): 1–12. For more on positive emotion and how it helps undo negative emotion, see B. L. Fredrickson, "The Role of Positive Emotions in Positive Psychology: The Broaden-and-Build Theory of Positive Emotions," *American Psychologist* 56, no. 3 (2001): 218–226, https://doi.org/10.1037/0003-066x.56.3.218.

34. For more on this study, see G. A. Bonanno, D. M. Colak, D. Keltner, M. N. Shiota, A. Papa, J. G. Noll, F. W. Putnam, and P. K. Trickett, "Context Matters: The Benefits and Costs of Expressing Positive Emotion Among Survivors of Childhood Sexual Abuse," *Emotion* 7, no. 4 (2007): 824–837, https:// doi.org/10.1037/1528-3542.7.4.824. For more on the consequences of disclosure of abuse, see D. Della Femina, C. A. Yeager, and D. O. Lewis, "Child Abuse: Adolescent Records vs. Adult Recall," *Child Abuse and Neglect* 14, no. 2 (1990): 227–231.

35. See E. B. Blanchard, E. J. Hickling, N. Mitnick, A. E. Taylor, W. R. Loos, and T. C. Buckley, "The Impact of Severity of Physical Injury and Perception of Life Threat in the Development of Post-Traumatic Stress Disorder in Motor Vehicle Accident Victims," *Behaviour Research and Therapy* 33, no. 5 (1995): 529–534, https://doi.org/10.1016/0005-7967(94)00079-Y; L. Meli, J. Birk, D. Edmondson, and G. A. Bonanno, "Trajectories of Posttraumatic Stress in Patients with Confirmed and Rule-Out Acute Coronary Syndrome," *General Hospital Psychiatry* 62 (2020): 37–42, https://doi.org/10.1016/j.genhosppsych.2019.11.006.

36. See T. L. Holbrook, D. B. Hoyt, M. B. Stein, and W. J. Sieber, "Perceived Threat to Life Predicts Posttraumatic Stress Disorder After Major Trauma: Risk Factors and Functional Outcome," *Journal of Trauma and Acute Care Surgery* 51, no. 2 (2001). For the 9/11 research, see G. A. Bonanno, C. Rennicke, and S. Dekel, "Self-Enhancement Among High-Exposure Survivors of the September

11th Terrorist Attack: Resilience or Social Maladjustment?," *Journal of Personality and Social Psychology* 88, no. 6 (2005): 984–998. See also C. N. Dulmus and C. Hilarski, "When Stress Constitutes Trauma and Trauma Constitutes Crisis: The Stress-Trauma-Crisis Continuum," *Brief Treatment and Crisis Intervention* 3, no. 1 (2003): 27–36.

37. For readable summaries of some of this work, see also Paul Slovic, "The Perception of Risk," in *Scientists Making a Difference: One Hundred Eminent Behavioral and Brain Scientists Talk About Their Most Important Contributions*, ed. Robert J. Sternberg, Susan T. Fiske, and Donald J. Foss, 179–182 (Cambridge: Cambridge University Press, 2016); V. J. Brown, "Risk Perception: It's Personal," *Environmental Health Perspectives* 122, no. 10 (2014): A276–A279, https://doi.org/10.1289 /ehp.122-A276. For more detailed scholarly papers on non-expert risk perception, see P. Slovic, "Perception of Risk," *Science* 236, no. 4799 (1987): 280–285, https://doi.org/10.1126/science.3563507; P. Slovic, ed., *The Feeling of Risk: New Perspectives on Risk Perception* (New York: Earthscan, 2010); G. F. Loewenstein, E. U. Weber, C. K. Hsee, and N. Welch, "Risk as Feelings," *Psychological Bulletin* 127, no. 2 (2001): 267–286, https://doi.org/10.1037/0033-2909.127.2.267.

38. Terri L. Messman-Moore and Selime R. Salim, "Risk Perception and Sexual Assault," in *Handbook of Sexual Assault and Sexual Assault Prevention*, ed. William T. O'Donohue and Paul A. Schewe, 211–228 (Cham, Switzerland: Springer, 2019), 211, https://doi.org/10.1007/978-3-030-23645-8_12.

39. A. E. Wilson, K. S. Calhoun, and J. A. Bernat, "Risk Recognition and Trauma-Related Symptoms Among Sexually Revictimized Women," *Journal of Consulting and Clinical Psychology* 67, no. 5 (1999): 705.

40. T. L. Messman-Moore and A. L. Brown, "Risk Perception, Rape, and Sexual Revictimization: A Prospective Study of College Women," *Psychology of Women Quarterly* 30, no. 2 (2006): 159–172.

41. See R. A. Ferrer, W. M. P. Klein, A. Avishai, K. Jones, M. Villegas, and P. Sheeran, "When Does Risk Perception Predict Protection Motivation for Health Threats? A Person-by-Situation Analysis," *PLoS ONE* 13, no. 3 (2018): e0191994–e0191994, https://doi.org/10.1371/journal.pone.0191994; M. Caserotti, E. Rubaltelli, and P. Slovic, "How Decision Context Changes the Balance Between Cost and Benefit Increasing Charitable Donations," *Judgment and Decision Making* 14, no. 2 (2019): 187–199; P. D. Windschitl and E. U. Weber, "The Interpretation of 'Likely' Depends on the Context, but '70%' Is 70%—Right? The Influence of Associative Processes on Perceived Certainty," *Journal of Experimental Psychology: Learning, Memory, and Cognition* 25, no. 6 (1999): 1514.

42. R. Goodwin, M. Willson, and G. Stanley Jr., "Terror Threat Perception and Its Consequences in Contemporary Britain," *British Journal of Psychology* 96, no. 4 (2005): 389–406.

43. I. R. Galatzer-Levy, M. M. Steenkamp, A. D. Brown, M. Qian, S. Inslicht, C. Henn-Haase, C. Otte, R. Yehuda, T. C. Neylan, and C. R. Marmar, "Cortisol Response to an Experimental Stress Paradigm Prospectively Predicts Long-Term Distress and Resilience Trajectories in Response to Active Police Service,"

Journal of Psychiatric Research 56 (2014): 36–42, https://doi.org/10.1016/j
.jpsychires.2014.04.020.

44. I. Wald, T. Shechner, S. Bitton, Y. Holoshitz, D. S. Charney, D. Muller,
N. A. Fox, D. S. Pine, and Y. Bar-Haim, "Attention Bias Away from Threat During
Life Threatening Danger Predicts PTSD Symptoms at One-Year Follow-Up,"
Depression and Anxiety 28, no. 5 (2011): 406–411, https://doi.org/10.1002/da
.20808. See also Y. Bar-Haim, D. Lamy, L. Pergamin, M. J. Bakermans-
Kranenburg, and M. H. van IJzendoorn, "Threat-Related Attentional Bias in
Anxious and Nonanxious Individuals: A Meta-Analytic Study," *Psychological Bul-
letin* 133 (2007): 1–24, https://doi.org/10.1037/0033-2909.133.1.1.

45. See L. Meli et al., "Trajectories of Posttraumatic Stress in Patients with
Confirmed and Rule-Out Acute Coronary Syndrome."

Chapter 5: A Mindset for Flexibility

1. Quote from C. Dweck, "What Having a 'Growth Mindset' Actually Means,"
Harvard Business Review 13 (2016): 213–226. For more on the growth mindset,
see also C. Dweck, "Carol Dweck Revisits the Growth Mindset," *Education Week*
35, no. 5 (2015): 20–24; Carol S. Dweck, *Mindset: The New Psychology of Success*
(New York: Random House, 2008).

2. See S. C. Kobasa, "Stressful Life Events, Personality, and Health: An Inquiry into Hardiness," *Journal of Personality and Social Psychology* 37, no. 1 (1979):
1–11.

3. S. C. Funk, "Hardiness: A Review of Theory and Research," *Health Psychology* 11 (1992): 335–345, https://doi.org/10.1037/0278-6133.11.5.335.

4. Kobasa, "Stressful Life Events"; S. R. Maddi, "Hardiness: The Courage
to Grow from Stresses," *Journal of Positive Psychology* 1, no. 3 (2006): 160–168
(quote from 160); V. Florian, M. Mikulincer, and O. Taubman, "Does Hardiness
Contribute to Mental Health During a Stressful Real-Life Situation? The Roles
of Appraisal and Coping," *Journal of Personality and Social Psychology* 68, no. 4
(1995): 687.

5. There are some key differences between the hardiness concept and the flexibility mindset. One of the original proponents of hardiness, Salvador Maddi,
went to pains to emphasize the nuanced characteristics of these components and
their distinctions from analogous concepts, including, for example, optimism.
See S. R. Maddi and M. Hightower, "Hardiness and Optimism as Expressed in
Coping Patterns," *Consulting Psychology Journal: Practice and Research* 51 (1999):
95–105, https://doi.org/10.1037/1061-4087.51.2.95. Maddi also argued that all
three components of hardiness are essential and that it is "insufficient to have only
one, or even two, of the hardy attitudes." I think of the flexibility mindset in more
general terms. The specific components are less crucial than the overall mindset.

6. M. F. Scheier, C. S. Carver, and M. W. Bridges, "Distinguishing Optimism from Neuroticism (and Trait Anxiety, Self-Mastery, and Self-Esteem): A

Reevaluation of the Life Orientation Test," *Journal of Personality and Social Psychology* 67, no. 6 (1994): 1063–1078; M. F. Scheier and C. S. Carver, "Optimism, Coping, and Health: Assessment and Implications of Generalized Outcome Expectancies," *Health Psychology* 4, no. 3 (1985): 219.

7. Emily Esfahani Smith, "The Benefits of Optimism Are Real," *The Atlantic*, March 1, 2013, www.theatlantic.com/health/archive/2013/03/the-benefits-of-optimism-are-real/273306; Steven M. Southwick and Dennis S. Charney, *Resilience: The Science of Mastering Life's Greatest Challenges* (Cambridge: Cambridge University Press, 2012); Martin E. P. Seligman, *Learned Optimism: How to Change Your Mind and Your Life* (New York: Vintage, 2012).

8. For example, see W. W. T. Lam, G. A. Bonanno, A. D. Mancini, S. Ho, M. Chan, W. K. Hung, A. Or, and R. Fielding, "Trajectories of Psychological Distress Among Chinese Women Diagnosed with Breast Cancer," *Psycho-Oncology* 19, no. 10 (2010): 1044–1051, https://doi.org/10.1002/pon.1658; F. Segovia, J. L. Moore, S. E. Linnville, R. E. Hoyt, and R. E. Hain, "Optimism Predicts Resilience in Repatriated Prisoners of War: A 37-Year Longitudinal Study," *Journal of Traumatic Stress* 25, no. 3 (2012): 330–336; A. J. Quale and A. K. Schanke, "Resilience in the Face of Coping with a Severe Physical Injury: A Study of Trajectories of Adjustment in a Rehabilitation Setting," *Rehabilitation Psychology* 55, no. 1 (2010): 12–22. For prospective findings, see I. R. Galatzer-Levy and G. A. Bonanno, "Optimism and Death: Predicting the Course and Consequences of Depression Trajectories in Response to Heart Attack," *Psychological Science* 25, no. 12 (2014): 2177–2188, https://doi.org/10.1177/0956797614551750. For a review of this research, see G. A. Bonanno, M. Westphal, and A. D. Mancini, "Resilience to Loss and Potential Trauma," *Annual Review of Clinical Psychology* 7 (2011), https://doi.org/10.1146/annurev-clinpsy-032210-104526.

9. See H. N. Rasmussen, M. F. Scheier, and J. B. Greenhouse, "Optimism and Physical Health: A Meta-Analytic Review," *Annals of Behavioral Medicine* 37, no. 3 (2009): 239–256, https://doi.org/10.1007/s12160-009-9111-x.

10. For examples of optimism failing to meaningfully predict better outcomes, see Y. Benyamini and I. Roziner, "The Predictive Validity of Optimism and Affectivity in a Longitudinal Study of Older Adults," *Personality and Individual Differences* 44, no. 4 (2008): 853–864, https://doi.org/10.1016/j.paid.2007.10.016; A. Serlachius, L. Pulkki-Råback, M. Elovainio, M. Hintsanen, V. Mikkilä, T. T. Laitinen, M. Jokela, et al., "Is Dispositional Optimism or Dispositional Pessimism Predictive of Ideal Cardiovascular Health? The Young Finns Study," *Psychology and Health* 30, no. 10 (2015): 1221–1239; E. Schoen, E. M. Altmaier, and B. Tallman, "Coping After Bone Marrow Transplantation: The Predictive Roles of Optimism and Dispositional Coping," *Journal of Clinical Psychology in Medical Settings* 14, no. 2 (2007): 123–129; H. I. M. Mahler and J. A. Kulik, "Optimism, Pessimism and Recovery from Coronary Bypass Surgery: Prediction of Affect, Pain and Functional Status," *Psychology, Health and Medicine* 5, no. 4 (2000): 347–358; K. R. Fontaine and L. C. Jones, "Self-Esteem, Optimism, and Postpartum Depression," *Journal of Clinical Psychology* 53, no. 1 (1997): 59–63.

11. A. Craig, Y. Tran, and J. Middleton, "Psychological Morbidity and Spinal Cord Injury: A Systematic Review," *Spinal Cord* 47, no. 2 (2009): 108–114.

12. For a recent example of how music, in combination with positive suggestions, can help with pain management, see H. Nowak, N. Zech, S. Asmussen, T. Rahmel, M. Tryba, G. Oprea, L. Grause, et al., "Effect of Therapeutic Suggestions During General Anaesthesia on Postoperative Pain and Opioid Use: Multicentre Randomised Controlled Trial," *BMJ* 371, m4284 (2021), https://doi.org/10.1136/bmj.m4284.

13. For an illuminating history of how the medical world has viewed spinal cord injuries, see Roberta B. Trieschmann, *Spinal Cord Injuries: The Psychological, Social, and Vocational Adjustment* (New York: Pergamon Press, 1988), 68.

14. T. Sharot, A. M. Riccardi, C. M. Raio, and E. A. Phelps, "Neural Mechanisms Mediating Optimism Bias," *Nature* 450, no. 7166 (2007): 102–105, https://doi.org/10.1038/nature06280. See also A. Etkin, T. Egner, D. M. Peraza, E. R. Kandel, and J. Hirsch, "Resolving Emotional Conflict: A Role for the Rostral Anterior Cingulate Cortex in Modulating Activity in the Amygdala," *Neuron* 51, no. 6 (2006): 871–882, https://doi.org/10.1016/j.neuron.2006.07.029.

15. For more on the motivation consequences of optimism, see C. S. Carver and M. F. Scheier, "Dispositional Optimism," *Trends in Cognitive Sciences* 18, no. 6 (2014): 293–299, https://doi.org/10.1016/j.tics.2014.02.003. For the motivating effect of optimism even in animals, see R. Rygula, J. Golebiowska, J. Kregiel, J. Kubik, and P. Popik, "Effects of Optimism on Motivation in Rats," *Frontiers in Behavioral Neuroscience* 9 (2015): 32, https://doi.org/10.3389/fnbeh.2015.00032.

16. L. O. Lee, P. James, E. S. Zevon, E. S. Kim, C. Trudel-Fitzgerald, A. Spiro III, F. Grodstein, and L. D. Kubzansky, "Optimism Is Associated with Exceptional Longevity in 2 Epidemiologic Cohorts of Men and Women," *Proceedings of the National Academy of Sciences* (2019): 201900712, https://doi.org/10.1073/pnas.1900712116.

17. See C. S. Carver, M. F. Scheier, and S. C. Segerstrom, "Optimism," *Clinical Psychology Review* 30, no. 7 (2010): 879–889; Carver and Scheier, "Dispositional Optimism."

18. M. M. Adams and A. L. Hicks, "Spasticity After Spinal Cord Injury," *Spinal Cord* 43, no. 10 (2005): 577–586, https://doi.org/10.1038/sj.sc.3101757.

19. R. D. Pentz, M. White, R. D. Harvey, Z. L. Farmer, Y. Liu, C. Lewis, O. Dashevskaya, T. Owonikoko, and F. R. Khuri, "Therapeutic Misconception, Misestimation, and Optimism in Participants Enrolled in Phase 1 Trials," *Cancer* 118, no. 18 (2012): 4571–4578, https://doi.org/10.1002/cncr.27397.

20. See K. Sweeny and J. A. Shepperd, "The Costs of Optimism and the Benefits of Pessimism," *Emotion* 10, no. 5 (2010): 750; M. W. Gallagher, L. J. Long, A. Richardson, and J. M. D'Souza, "Resilience and Coping in Cancer Survivors: The Unique Effects of Optimism and Mastery," *Cognitive Therapy and Research* 43, no. 1 (2019): 32–44; M. Cohen, I. Levkovich, S. Pollack, and G. Fried, "Stability and Change of Post-Chemotherapy Symptoms in Relation to Optimism

and Subjective Stress: A Prospective Study of Breast Cancer Survivors," *Psycho-Oncology* 28, no. 10 (2019): 2017–2024.

21. Gerald G. Jampolsky, *Teach Only Love: The Seven Principles of Attitudinal Healing* (New York: Bantam Books, 1983).

Chapter 6: Synergy

1. G. A. Bonanno, "Identity Continuity and Complexity in Resilience and Recovery from Loss," *Making Sense of the Unimaginable: How Meaning Making Dynamics Shape Recovery from Severe Stress Experiences*, symposium, E. de St. Aubin, chair, at the Association for Psychological Science 20th Annual Convention, Chicago, 2008.

2. G. A. Bonanno, P. Kennedy, I. Galatzer-Levy, P. Lude, and M. L. Elfström, "Trajectories of Resilience, Depression, and Anxiety Following Spinal Cord Injury," *Rehabilitation Psychology* 57, no. 3 (2012): 236–247; A. Craig, Y. Tran, and J. Middleton, "Psychological Morbidity and Spinal Cord Injury: A Systematic Review," *Spinal Cord* 47, no. 2 (2009): 108–114; K. M. Hancock, A. R. Craig, H. G. Dickson, E. Chang, and J. Martin, "Anxiety and Depression over the First Year of Spinal Cord Injury: A Longitudinal Study," *Spinal Cord* 31, no. 6 (1993): 349–357.

3. See O. Vassend, A. J. Quale, O. Røise, and A.-K. Schanke, "Predicting the Long-Term Impact of Acquired Severe Injuries on Functional Health Status: The Role of Optimism, Emotional Distress and Pain," *Spinal Cord* 49, no. 12 (2011): 1193–1197, https://doi.org/10.1038/sc.2011.70; B. Akbari, S. F. Shahkhali, and R. G. Jobaneh, "Canonical Analysis of the Relationships of Religiosity, Hope, and Optimism with the Meaning of Life and Quality of Life in Spinal Cord Injury Patients," *Journal of Religion and Health* 7, no. 1 (2019): 11–19; Bonanno et al., "Trajectories of Resilience"; K. P. Arbour-Nicitopoulos, K. A. M. Ginis, and A. E. Latimer, "Planning, Leisure-Time Physical Activity, and Confidence in Coping in Persons with Spinal Cord Injury: A Randomized Controlled Trial," *Archives of Physical Medicine and Rehabilitation* 90, no. 12 (2009): 2003–2011, https://doi.org/10.1016/j.apmr.2009.06.019; I. R. Molton, M. P. Jensen, W. Nielson, D. Cardenas, and D. M. Ehde, "A Preliminary Evaluation of the Motivational Model of Pain Self-Management in Persons with Spinal Cord Injury-Related Pain," *Journal of Pain* 9, no. 7 (2008): 606–612, https://doi.org/10.1016/j.jpain.2008.01.338.

4. See A. Bandura, D. Cioffi, C. B. Taylor, and M. E. Brouillard, "Perceived Self-Efficacy in Coping with Cognitive Stressors and Opioid Activation," *Journal of Personality and Social Psychology* 55, no. 3 (1988): 479–488, https://doi.org/10.1037/0022-3514.55.3.479; C. Cozzarelli, "Personality and Self-Efficacy as Predictors of Coping with Abortion," *Journal of Personality and Social Psychology* 65, no. 6 (1993): 1224–1236, https://doi.org/10.1037/0022-3514.65.6.1224; E. J. Philip, T. V. Merluzzi, Z. Zhang, and C. A. Heitzmann, "Depression and

Cancer Survivorship: Importance of Confidence in Coping in Post-Treatment Survivors," *Psycho-Oncology* 22, no. 5 (2013): 987–994, https://doi.org/10.1002 /pon.3088; J. A. Turner, M. Ersek, and C. Kemp, "Self-Efficacy for Managing Pain Is Associated with Disability, Depression, and Pain Coping Among Retirement Community Residents with Chronic Pain," *Journal of Pain* 6, no. 7 (2005): 471–479, https://doi.org/10.1016/j.jpain.2005.02.011; M. W. G. Bosmans, H. W. Hofland, A. E. De Jong, and N. E. Van Loey, "Coping with Burns: The Role of Confidence in Coping in the Recovery from Traumatic Stress Following Burn Injuries," *Journal of Behavioral Medicine* 38, no. 4 (2015): 642–651, https://doi.org/10.1007/s10865-015-9638-1; M. W. G. Bosmans and P. G. van der Velden, "Longitudinal Interplay Between Posttraumatic Stress Symptoms and Confidence in Coping: A Four-Wave Prospective Study," *Social Science and Medicine* 134 (2015): 23–29, https://doi.org/10.1016/j.socscimed.2015.04.007; C. Benight and M. Harper, "Confidence in Coping Perceptions as a Mediator Between Acute Stress Response and Long-Term Distress Following Natural Disasters," *Journal of Traumatic Stress* 15 (2002): 177–186, https://doi.org /10.1023/A:1015295025950.

5. T. A. DeRoon-Cassini, A. D. Mancini, M. D. Rusch, and G. A. Bonanno, "Psychopathology and Resilience Following Traumatic Injury: A Latent Growth Mixture Model Analysis," *Rehabilitation Psychology* 55, no. 1 (2010): 1–11, https://doi.org/10.1037/a0018601. See also M. E. Wadsworth, C. D. Santiago, and L. Einhorn, "Coping with Displacement from Hurricane Katrina: Predictors of One-Year Post-Traumatic Stress and Depression Symptom Trajectories," *Anxiety, Stress, and Coping* 22, no. 4 (2009): 413–432, https://doi.org /10.1080/10615800902855781.

6. J. Tomaka, J. Blascovich, J. Kibler, and J. M. Ernst, "Cognitive and Physiological Antecedents of Threat and Challenge Appraisal," *Journal of Personality and Social Psychology* 73 (1997): 63–72.

7. Nate Chinen, "As a Crowdfunding Platform Implodes, a Legendary Composer Rebounds," NPR, May 14, 2019, www.npr.org/2019/05/14/723225435 /as-a-crowdfunding-platform-implodes-a-legendary-composer-rebounds.

8. Tomaka et al., "Cognitive and Physiological Antecedents."

9. J. Gaab, N. Rohleder, U. M. Nater, and U. Ehlert, "Psychological Determinants of the Cortisol Stress Response: The Role of Anticipatory Cognitive Appraisal," *Psychoneuroendocrinology* 30, no. 6 (2005): 599–610, https://doi .org/10.1016/j.psyneuen.2005.02.001; A. Harvey, A. B. Nathens, G. Bandiera, and V. R. LeBlanc, "Threat and Challenge: Cognitive Appraisal and Stress Responses in Simulated Trauma Resuscitations," *Medical Education* 44, no. 6 (2010): 587–594, https://doi.org/10.1111/j.1365-2923.2010.03634.x; K. Maier, S. Waldstein, and S. Synowski, "Relation of Cognitive Appraisal to Cardiovascular Reactivity, Affect, and Task Engagement," *Annals of Behavioral Medicine* 26, no. 1 (2003): 32–41, https://doi.org/10.1207/S15324796ABM2601_05.

10. Jim Blascovich and Wendy Berry Mendes, "Challenge and Threat Appraisals: The Role of Affective Cues," in *Feeling and Thinking: The Role of Affect in Social*

Cognition, ed. Joseph P. Forgas, 59–82 (Cambridge: Cambridge University Press, 2000).

11. S. C. Hunter, J. M. E. Boyle, and D. Warden, "Help Seeking Amongst Child and Adolescent Victims of Peer-Aggression and Bullying: The Influence of School-Stage, Gender, Victimisation, Appraisal, and Emotion," *British Journal of Educational Psychology* 74, no. 3 (2004): 375–390, https://doi.org/10.1348/0007099041552378; J. M. Schaubroeck, L. T. Riolli, A. C. Peng, and E. S. Spain, "Resilience to Traumatic Exposure Among Soldiers Deployed in Combat," *Journal of Occupational Health Psychology* 16, no. 1 (2011): 18–37, https://doi.org/10.1037/a0021006.

12. Paul Kennedy told me the bricklayer story one night over dinner. The story is also mentioned in Gary Marcus, "Dancing Without Feet," *New Yorker*, March 23, 2013, www.newyorker.com/culture/culture-desk/dancing-without-feet.

13. P. Kennedy, M. Evans, and N. Sandhu, "Psychological Adjustment to Spinal Cord Injury: The Contribution of Coping, Hope and Cognitive Appraisals," *Psychology, Health and Medicine* 14, no. 1 (2009): 17–33, https://doi.org/10.1080/13548500802001801.

14. Bonanno et al., "Trajectories of Resilience."

15. M. L. Elfström, A. Rydén, M. Kreuter, L.-O. Persson, and M. Sullivan, "Linkages Between Coping and Psychological Outcome in the Spinal Cord Lesioned: Development of SCL-Related Measures," *Spinal Cord* 40, no. 1 (2002): 23–29, https://doi.org/10.1038/sj.sc.3101238.

16. See P. Schönfeld, F. Preusser, and J. Margraf, "Costs and Benefits of Self-Efficacy: Differences of the Stress Response and Clinical Implications," *Neuroscience and Biobehavioral Reviews* 75 (2017): 40–52, https://doi.org/10.1016/j.neubiorev.2017.01.031; A. A. Nease, B. O. Mudgett, and M. A. Quiñones, "Relationships Among Feedback Sign, Self-Efficacy, and Acceptance of Performance Feedback," *Journal of Applied Psychology* 84, no. 5 (1999): 806; E. S. Epel, B. S. McEwen, and J. R. Ickovics, "Embodying Psychological Thriving: Physical Thriving in Response to Stress," *Journal of Social Issues* 54 (1998): 301–322.

17. See C. C. Benight, E. Swift, J. Sanger, A. Smith, and D. Zeppelin, "Confidence in Coping as a Mediator of Distress Following a Natural Disaster," *Journal of Applied Social Psychology* 29, no. 12 (1999): 2443–2464, https://doi.org/10.1111/j.1559-1816.1999.tb00120; I. Levkovich, M. Cohen, S. Pollack, K. Drumea, and G. Fried, "Cancer-Related Fatigue and Depression in Breast Cancer Patients Postchemotherapy: Different Associations with Optimism and Stress Appraisals," *Palliative and Supportive Care* 13, no. 5 (2015): 1141–1151.

18. R. Delahaij and K. Van Dam, "Coping with Acute Stress in the Military: The Influence of Coping Style, Coping Self-Efficacy and Appraisal Emotions," *Personality and Individual Differences* 119 (2017): 13–18, https://doi.org/10.1016/j.paid.2017.06.021.

19. Matthias Jerusalem and Ralf Schwarzer, "Self-Efficacy as a Resource Factor in Stress Appraisal Processes," in *Self-Efficacy: Thought Control of Action*, ed. Ralf Schwarzer, 195–213 (New York: Taylor and Francis, 1992); M. A. Chesney,

T. B. Neilands, D. B. Chambers, J. M. Taylor, and S. Folkman, "A Validity and Reliability Study of the Coping Self-Efficacy Scale," *British Journal of Health Psychology* 11, no. 3 (2006): 421–437.

20. S. Chen and T. Jackson, "Causal Effects of Challenge and Threat Appraisals on Pain Self-Efficacy, Pain Coping, and Tolerance for Laboratory Pain: An Experimental Path Analysis Study," *PLoS ONE* 14, no. 4 (2019): e0215087, https://doi.org/10.1371/journal.pone.0215087. See also N. Skinner and N. Brewer, "The Dynamics of Threat and Challenge Appraisals Prior to Stressful Achievement Events," *Journal of Personality and Social Psychology* 83, no. 3 (2002): 678; E. C. Karademas, "Self-Efficacy, Social Support and Well-Being: The Mediating Role of Optimism," *Personality and Individual Differences* 40, no. 6 (2006): 1281–1290, https://doi.org/10.1016/j.paid.2005.10.019.

21. Hayden Herrera, *Frida: A Biography of Frida Kahlo* (New York: Harper and Row, 1983).

22. Herrera, *Frida*, 48.

23. Herrera, *Frida*, 49.

24. Frida Kahlo, *The Letters of Frida Kahlo: Cartas Apasionadas*, ed. Martha Zamora (San Francisco: Chronicle, 1995), 22.

25. Salomon Grimberg, *Frida Kahlo: Song of Herself* (London: Merrell, 2008).

26. Herrera, *Frida*; Grimberg, *Frida Kahlo*.

27. Herrera, *Frida*, 65.

28. Herrera, *Frida*.

29. Grimberg, *Frida Kahlo*, 65.

30. Herrera, *Frida*.

31. Grimberg, *Frida Kahlo*, 65–67.

32. Herrera, *Frida*, 63.

33. Grimberg, *Frida Kahlo*.

34. Diego Rivera, *My Art, My Life* (New York: Citadel, 1960), 103–104.

35. Rivera, *My Art, My Life*, 104.

36. J. Helland, "Aztec Imagery in Frida Kahlo's Paintings: Indigenity and Political Commitment," *Woman's Art Journal* 11, no. 2 (1990): 8–13, https://doi.org/10.2307/3690692; Grimberg, *Frida Kahlo*, 33–34.

37. Frida Kahlo, *The Diary of Frida Kahlo: An Intimate Self-Portrait*, with an introduction by Carlos Fuentes and essay and commentaries by Sarah M. Lowe (New York: Harry N. Abrams, 2005), 252.

38. Grimberg, *Frida Kahlo*, 105.

39. Quote from the documentary film *The Life and Times of Frida Kahlo*, written and directed by Amy Stechler, a production of Daylight Films and WETA in association with Latino Public Broadcasting, PBS Home Video, 2005.

40. Quote from "Mexican Autobiography," *Time* 61, no. 17 (1953): 90.

41. Quote from *Life and Times of Frida Kahlo*.

42. Quoted in Daniel Bullen, *The Love Lives of the Artists: Five Stories of Creative Intimacy* (Berkeley, CA: Counterpoint, 2013).

43. Herrera, *Frida*, 416.

44. Herrera, *Frida*, 419; Carole Maso, *Beauty Is Convulsive: The Passion of Frida Kahlo* (Washington, DC: Counterpoint, 2002), 146.

45. Frida Kahlo Museum, also known as La Casa Azul (The Blue House), Mexico City.

46. Herrera, *Frida*, 75.

47. Herrera, *Frida*, 75.

48. Herrera, *Frida*, 142.

49. Herrera, *Frida*, 142.

50. Kahlo, *Diary*, 274.

Chapter 7: The Flexibility Sequence

1. Thanks to my colleagues June Gruber, Iris Mauss, and Maya Tamir for pointing to Aristotle in their paper "A Dark Side of Happiness? How, When, and Why Happiness Is Not Always Good," *Perspectives on Psychological Science* 6, no. 3 (2011): 222–233, https://doi.org/10.1177/1745691611406927. Although translations vary, my source for the quote was *Nicomachean Ethics*, trans. H. Rachman, (Cambridge, MA: Harvard University Press, 1936), Book 2, chap. 9.

2. Seneca, "On the Tranquility of the Mind," in *Seneca: Dialogues and Essays*, ed. J. Davie and T. Reinhardt (New York: Oxford University Press, 2007), 133.

3. See J. Rottenberg, J. J. Gross, and I. H. Gotlib, "Emotion Context Insensitivity in Major Depressive Disorder," *Journal of Abnormal Psychology* 114, no. 4 (2005): 627–639, https://doi.org/10.1037/0021-843X.114.4.627; K. G. Coifman and G. A. Bonanno, "When Distress Does Not Become Depression: Emotion Context Sensitivity and Adjustment to Bereavement," *Journal of Abnormal Psychology* 119, no. 3 (2010): 479–490, https://doi.org/10.1037/a0020113.

4. G. A. Bonanno, F. Maccallum, M. Malgaroli, and W. K. Hou, "The Context Sensitivity Index (CSI): Measuring the Ability to Identify the Presence and Absence of Stressor Context Cues," *Assessment* 27, no. 2 (2020), https://doi.org/10.1177/1073191118820131.

5. See Coifman and Bonanno, "When Distress Does Not Become Depression."

6. S. Folkman and R. S. Lazarus, "If It Changes It Must Be a Process: Study of Emotion and Coping During Three Stages of a College Examination," *Journal of Personality and Social Psychology* 48, no. 1 (1985): 150–170, https://doi.org/10.1037/0022-3514.48.1.150; A. M. Malooly, J. J. Genet, and M. Siemer, "Individual Differences in Reappraisal Effectiveness: The Role of Affective Flexibility," *Emotion* 13, no. 2 (2013): 302.

7. E. Levy-Gigi, C. Szabo, G. Richter-Levin, and S. Kéri, "Reduced Hippocampal Volume Is Associated with Overgeneralization of Negative Context in Individuals with PTSD," *Neuropsychology* 29, no. 1 (2015): 151.

8. Psychologists who study goals have learned that most of us organize our personal goals hierarchically, from concrete, short-term, context-dependent goals to more abstract, enduring, and long-term or superordinate goals. Most people

typically rely on several interrelated goal hierarches. But within these hierarchies, superordinate goals are generally more important personally, while lower-order goals that help satisfy superordinate goals are generally viewed as more important than lower-order goals that do not. For more on goal hierarchies, see H. N. Rasmussen, C. Wrosch, M. F. Scheier, and C. S. Carver, "Self-Regulation Processes and Health: The Importance of Optimism and Goal Adjustment," *Journal of Personality* 74, no. 6 (2006): 1721–1748. See also A. Duckworth and J. J. Gross, "Self-Control and Grit: Related but Separable Determinants of Success," *Current Directions in Psychological Science* 23, no. 5 (2014): 319–325, https://doi .org/10.1177/0963721414541462.

9. E. A. Skinner and M. J. Zimmer-Gembeck, "The Development of Coping," *Annual Review of Psychology* 48 (2007): 119–144.

10. See J. E. Heiy and J. S. Cheavens, "Back to Basics: A Naturalistic Assessment of the Experience and Regulation of Emotion," *Emotion* 14, no. 5 (2014): 878; G. Grommisch, P. Koval, J. D. X. Hinton, J. Gleeson, T. Hollenstein, P. Kuppens, and T. Lischetzke, "Modeling Individual Differences in Emotion Regulation Repertoire in Daily Life with Multilevel Latent Profile Analysis," *Emotion* 20, no. 8 (2020): 1462–1474, https://doi.org/10.1037/emo0000669.

11. The experiment I developed was adapted from an earlier experiment to study emotional suppression developed by James Gross and Robert Levenson. See J. J. Gross and R. W. Levenson, "Emotional Suppression: Physiology, Self-Report, and Expressive Behavior," *Journal of Personality and Social Psychology* 64, no. 6 (1993): 970–986; J. J. Gross and R. W. Levenson, "Hiding Feelings: The Acute Effects of Inhibiting Negative and Positive Emotion," *Journal of Abnormal Psychology* 106, no. 1 (1997): 95–103. For more details on how I adapted this task, see G. A. Bonanno, A. Papa, K. Lalande, M. Westphal, and K. Coifman, "The Importance of Being Flexible: The Ability to Both Enhance and Suppress Emotional Expression Predicts Long-Term Adjustment," *Psychological Science* 15, no. 7 (2004): 482–487.

12. Bonanno et al., "The Importance of Being Flexible."

13. See C. L. Burton and G. A. Bonanno, "Measuring Ability to Enhance and Suppress Emotional Expression: The Flexible Regulation of Emotional Expression (FREE) Scale," *Psychological Assessment* 28, no. 8 (2016): 929–941, https://doi .org/10.1037/pas0000231.

14. See C. Cheng, "Assessing Coping Flexibility in Real-Life and Laboratory Settings: A Multimethod Approach," *Journal of Personality and Social Psychology* 80, no. 5 (2001): 814–833. For a broad review of this research, see C. Cheng, H.-P. B. Lau, and M.-P. S. Chan, "Coping Flexibility and Psychological Adjustment to Stressful Life Changes: A Meta-Analytic Review," *Psychological Bulletin* 140, no. 6 (2014): 1582–1607, https://doi.org/10.1037/a0037913. In addition, see G. A. Bonanno, R. Pat-Horenczyk, and J. Noll, "Coping Flexibility and Trauma: The Perceived Ability to Cope with Trauma (PACT) Scale," *Psychological Trauma-Theory Research Practice and Policy* 3, no. 2 (2011): 117–129, https://doi

.org/10.1037/a0020921; M. Park, E. R. Chang, and S. You, "Protective Role of Coping Flexibility in PTSD and Depressive Symptoms Following Trauma," *Personality and Individual Differences* 82 (2015): 102–106, https://doi.org/10.1016 /j.paid.2015.03.007; I. R. Galatzer-Levy, C. L. Burton, and G. A. Bonanno, "Coping Flexibility, Potentially Traumatic Life Events, and Resilience: A Prospective Study of College Student Adjustment," *Journal of Social and Clinical Psychology* 31, no. 6 (2012): 542–567, https://doi.org/10.1521/jscp.2012.31.6.542; C. L. Burton, O. H. Yan, R. Pat-Horenczyk, I. S. F. Chan, S. Ho, and G. A. Bonanno, "Coping Flexibility and Complicated Grief: A Comparison of American and Chinese Samples," *Depression and Anxiety* 29, no. 1 (2012): 16–22, https://doi .org/10.1002/da.20888; R. Rodin, G. A. Bonanno, S. Knuckey, M. L. Satter-thwaite, R. Hart, A. Joscelyne, R. A. Bryant, and A. D. Brown, "Coping Flexibility Predicts Post-Traumatic Stress Disorder and Depression in Human Rights Advocates," *International Journal of Mental Health* 46, no. 4 (2017): 327–338, https://doi.org/10.1080/00207411.2017.1345047; G. Boyraz, M. L. Cherry, M. A. Cherry, S. Aarstad-Martin, C. Cloud, and L. M. Shamp, "Posttraumatic Stress, Coping Flexibility, and Risky Drinking Among Trauma-Exposed Male and Female College Students: The Mediating Effect of Delay of Gratification," *Substance Use and Misuse* 53, no. 3 (2018): 508–520.

15. See R. E. Morgan and B. A. Oudekerk, "Criminal Victimization, 2018," US Department of Justice, Bureau of Justice Statistics, September 2019, www.bjs .gov/content/pub/pdf/cv18.pdf; S. Bricknell, H. Boxall, and H. Andrevski, *Male Victims of Non-Sexual and Non-Domestic Violence: Service Needs and Experiences in Court*, Australian Institute of Criminology, Research and Public Policy Series, vol. 126, 2014, available at https://aic.gov.au/publications/rpp/rpp126.

16. See Morgan and Oudekerk, "Criminal Victimization, 2018"; D. Freeman, C. Thompson, N. Vorontsova, G. Dunn, L.-A. Carter, P. Garety, E. Kuipers, et al., "Paranoia and Post-Traumatic Stress Disorder in the Months After a Physical Assault: A Longitudinal Study Examining Shared and Differential Predictors," *Psychological Medicine* 43, no. 12 (2013): 2673–2684, https://doi.org/10.1017 /S003329171300038X; Bricknell et al., *Male Victims of Non-Sexual and Non-Domestic Violence*; V. Burcar, "Doing Masculinity in Narratives About Reporting Violent Crime: Young Male Victims Talk About Contacting and Encountering the Police," *Journal of Youth Studies* 16, no. 2 (2013): 172–190, https://doi .org/10.1080/13676261.2012.704992; Veronika Burcar, "Masculinity and Victimization: Young Men's Talk About Being Victims of Violent Crime," in *Masculinities in the Criminological Field: Control, Vulnerability and Risk-Taking*, ed. Ingrid Lander, Signe Ravn, and Nina Jon, 113–130 (London: Routledge, 2016).

17. For a readable summary of this work, see J. E. LeDoux, "Feelings: What Are They and How Does the Brain Make Them?," *Daedalus* 144, no. 1 (2015): 96–111. See also J. E. LeDoux and R. Brown, "A Higher-Order Theory of Emotional Consciousness," *Proceedings of the National Academy of Sciences* (2017), https:// doi.org/10.1073/pnas.1619316114; F. Rigoli, M. Ewbank, T. Dalgleish, and

A. Calder, "Threat Visibility Modulates the Defensive Brain Circuit Underlying Fear and Anxiety," *Neuroscience Letters* 612 (2016): 7–13, https://doi.org/10.1016/j.neulet.2015.11.026.

18. For more on fear and anxiety, see Ame Öhman, "Fear and Anxiety: Overlaps and Dissociations," in *Handbook of Emotions*, 3rd ed., ed. Michael Lewis, Jeannette M. Haviland-Jones, and Lisa Feldman Barrett, 709–729 (New York: Guilford Press, 2008); C. A. Hartley and E. A. Phelps, "Anxiety and Decision-Making," *Biological Psychiatry* 72, no. 2 (2012): 113–118, https://doi.org/10.1016/j.biopsych.2011.12.027; Y. Bar-Haim, A. Kerem, D. Lamy, and D. Zakay, "When Time Slows Down: The Influence of Threat on Time Perception in Anxiety," *Cognition and Emotion* 24, no. 2 (2010): 255–263, https://doi.org/10.1080/02699930903387603.

19. We also explored the opposite pattern, asking participants to begin with distraction and then giving them the opportunity to switch to reappraisal. However, because reappraisal tends not to work well, and people tend not to use it when emotions are extreme or intense, we did not observe a clear pattern of switching to this strategy. For more on these studies, see J. L. Birk and G. A. Bonanno, "When to Throw the Switch: The Adaptiveness of Modifying Emotion Regulation Strategies Based on Affective and Physiological Feedback," *Emotion* 16, no. 5 (2016): 657–670. For a related experimental study, see S. D. Ilan, R. Shafir, J. L. Birk, G. A. Bonanno, and G. Sheppes, "Monitoring in Emotion Regulation: Behavioral Decisions and Neural Consequences," *Social Cognitive and Affective Neuroscience* 1 (2020): 1–11. For related nonexperimental evidence, see T. Kato, "Development of the Coping Flexibility Scale: Evidence for the Coping Flexibility Hypothesis," *Journal of Counseling Psychology* 59, no. 2 (2012): 262–273, https://doi.org/10.1037/a0027770; T. Kato, "Testing of the Coping Flexibility Hypothesis Based on the Dual-Process Theory: Relationships Between Coping Flexibility and Depressive Symptoms," *Psychiatry Research* 230, no. 2 (2015): 137–142, https://doi.org/10.1016/j.psychres.2015.07.030.

20. Ilan et al., "Monitoring in Emotion Regulation," 11.

21. See J. S. Beer, E. A. Heerey, D. Keltner, D. Scabini, and R. T. Knight, "The Regulatory Function of Self-Conscious Emotion: Insights from Patients with Orbitofrontal Damage," *Journal of Personality and Social Psychology* 85, no. 4 (2003): 594–604, https://doi.org/10.1037/0022-3514.85.4.594; A. Kitsantas, B. J. Zimmerman, and T. Cleary, "The Role of Observation and Emulation in the Development of Athletic Self-Regulation," *Journal of Educational Psychology* 92, no. 4 (2000): 811–817; C. G. Davey, N. B. Allen, B. J. Harrison, and M. Yücel, "Increased Amygdala Response to Positive Social Feedback in Young People with Major Depressive Disorder," *Biological Psychiatry* 69, no. 8 (2011): 734–741, https://doi.org/10.1016/j.biopsych.2010.12.004; Katherine A. Loveland, "Social-Emotional Impairment and Self-Regulation in Autism Spectrum," in *Emotional Development: Recent Research Advances*, ed. Jacqueline Nadel and Darwin Muir, 365–376 (Oxford: Oxford University Press, 2005).

22. For more on memory consolidation and reconsolidation, see R. Bisaz, A. Travaglia, and C. M. Alberini, "The Neurobiological Bases of Memory Formation: From Physiological Conditions to Psychopathology," *Psychopathology* 47, no. 6 (2014): 347–356, https://doi.org/10.1159/000363702; R. A. Bryant and S. Datta, "Reconsolidating Intrusive Distressing Memories by Thinking of Attachment Figures," *Clinical Psychological Science* 7, no. 6 (2019): 1249–1256, https://doi.org/10.1177/2167702619866387; D. Schiller, M.-H. Monfils, C. M. Raio, D. C. Johnson, J. E. LeDoux, and E. A. Phelps, "Preventing the Return of Fear in Humans Using Reconsolidation Update Mechanisms," *Nature* 463, no. 7277 (2010): 49–53; J. L. C. Lee, "Memory Reconsolidation Mediates the Strengthening of Memories by Additional Learning," *Nature Neuroscience* 11, no. 11 (2008): 1264.

23. S. Dekel and G. A. Bonanno, "Changes in Trauma Memory and Patterns of Posttraumatic Stress," *Psychological Trauma: Theory, Research, Practice, and Policy* 5, no. 1 (2013): 26–34, https://doi.org/10.1037/a0022750. For another example, see C. F. Weems, J. D. Russell, D. M. Banks, R. A. Graham, E. L. Neill, and B. G. Scott, "Memories of Traumatic Events in Childhood Fade After Experiencing Similar Less Stressful Events: Results from Two Natural Experiments," *Journal of Experimental Psychology: General* 143, no. 5 (2014): 2046–2055, https://doi .org/10.1037/xge0000016.

24. Bryant and Datta, "Reconsolidating Intrusive Distressing Memories."

25. S. Chen and G. A. Bonanno, "Components of Emotion Regulation Flexibility: Linking Latent Profiles to Symptoms of Depression and Anxiety," *Clinical Psychological Science* 9(2), 236–251 (2021), https://doi.org/10.1177/2167702 620956972.

Chapter 8: Becoming Flexible

1. Amy Wolf, "Why Does It Take Humans So Long to Mature Compared to Other Animals? Look to Your Neurons!," Vanderbilt University, https://news .vanderbilt.edu/2018/10/30/why-does-it-take-humans-so-long-to-mature -compared-to-other-animals-look-to-your-neurons. For more information on the published research, see S. Herculano-Houzel, "Longevity and Sexual Maturity Vary Across Species with Number of Cortical Neurons, and Humans Are No Exception," *Journal of Comparative Neurology* 527, no. 10 (2019): 1689–1705.

2. N. Emese, "Is Newborn Smiling Really Just a Reflex? Research Is Challenging Our Textbooks," *The Conversation*, n.d., https://theconversation.com/is -newborn-smiling-really-just-a-reflex-research-is-challenging-the-textbooks -105220. See also E. Nagy, "The Newborn Infant: A Missing Stage in Developmental Psychology," *Infant and Child Development* 20, no. 1 (2011): 3–19, https://doi .org/10.1002/icd.683.

3. See G. D. Heyman and B. J. Compton, "Context Sensitivity in Children's Reasoning About Ability Across the Elementary School Years," *Developmental*

Science 9, no. 6 (2006): 616–627; T. Imada, S. M. Carlson, and S. Itakura, "East–West Cultural Differences in Context-Sensitivity Are Evident in Early Childhood," *Developmental Science* 16, no. 2 (2013): 198–208; M. Köster, J. Castel, T. Gruber, and J. Kärtner, "Visual Cortical Networks Align with Behavioral Measures of Context-Sensitivity in Early Childhood," *NeuroImage* 163 (2017): 413–418, https://doi.org/10.1016/j.neuroimage.2017.08.008.

4. For more details on these studies, see W. F. Arsenio, S. Cooperman, and A. Lover, "Affective Predictors of Preschoolers' Aggression and Peer Acceptance: Direct and Indirect Effects," *Developmental Psychology* 36, no. 4 (2000): 438; K. A. Buss, R. J. Davidson, N. H. Kalin, and H. H. Goldsmith, "Context-Specific Freezing and Associated Physiological Reactivity as a Dysregulated Fear Response," *Developmental Psychology* 40, no. 4 (2004): 583.

5. For a review of this research, see E. A. Skinner and M. J. Zimmer-Gembeck, "The Development of Coping," *Annual Review of Psychology* 58 (2007): 119–144; K. A. Babb, L. J. Levine, and J. M. Arseneault, "Shifting Gears: Coping Flexibility in Children with and Without ADHD," *International Journal of Behavioral Development* 34, no. 1 (2010): 10–23; E. L. Davis, L. J. Levine, H. C. Lench, and J. A. Quas, "Metacognitive Emotion Regulation: Children's Awareness That Changing Thoughts and Goals Can Alleviate Negative Emotions," *Emotion* 10, no. 4 (2010): 498–510, https://doi.org/10.1037/a0018428.

6. For more on this research, see S. D. Espinet, J. E. Anderson, and P. D. Zelazo, "Reflection Training Improves Executive Function in Preschool-Age Children: Behavioral and Neural Effects," *Developmental Cognitive Neuroscience* 4 (2013): 3–15; P. D. Zelazo, "Executive Function: Reflection, Iterative Reprocessing, Complexity, and the Developing Brain," *Developmental Review* 38 (2015): 55–68; J. Shrager and R. S. Siegler, "SCADS: A Model of Children's Strategy Choices and Strategy Discoveries," *Psychological Science* 9, no. 5 (1998): 405–410; M. W. Alibali, "How Children Change Their Minds: Strategy Change Can Be Gradual or Abrupt," *Developmental Psychology* 35, no. 1 (1999): 127; Davis et al., "Metacognitive Emotion Regulation."

7. B. B. R. Rossman, "School-Age Children's Perceptions of Coping with Distress: Strategies for Emotion Regulation and the Moderation of Adjustment," *Journal of Child Psychology and Psychiatry* 33, no. 8 (1992): 1375.

8. B. E. Compas, J. K. Connor-Smith, H. Saltzman, A. H. Thomsen, and M. E. Wadsworth, "Coping with Stress During Childhood and Adolescence: Problems, Progress, and Potential in Theory and Research," *Psychological Bulletin* 127, no. 1 (2001): 87, 89.

9. There are a number of readable books on the vast and growing scientific literature on conscious and unconscious or nonconscious processes. For a particularly compelling review, I suggest Stanislas Dehaene, *Consciousness and the Brain: Deciphering How the Brain Codes Our Thoughts* (New York: Penguin, 2014).

10. See W. Schneider and R. M. Shiffrin, "Controlled and Automatic Human Information Processing: I. Detection, Search, and Attention," *Psychological Review* 84, no. 1 (1977): 1; R. M. Shiffrin and W. Schneider, "Controlled and Automatic

Human Information Processing: II. Perceptual Learning, Automatic Attending and a General Theory," *Psychological Review* 84, no. 2 (1977): 127.

11. A. G. Wheaton, D. P. Chapman, L. R. Presley-Cantrell, J. B. Croft, and D. R. Roehler, "Drowsy Driving-19 States and the District of Columbia, 2009–2010," *Morbidity and Mortality Weekly Report* 61, no. 51 (2013): 1033.

12. Heyman and Compton, "Context Sensitivity in Children's Reasoning About Ability."

13. For more information on these studies, see B. K. Payne, "Prejudice and Perception: The Role of Automatic and Controlled Processes in Misperceiving a Weapon," *Journal of Personality and Social Psychology* 81, no. 2 (2001): 181; B. K. Payne, A. J. Lambert, & L. L. Jacoby, (2002). "Best Laid Plans: Effects of Goals on Accessibility Bias and Cognitive Control in Race-Based Misperceptions of Weapons," *Journal of Experimental Social Psychology* 38, no. 4 (2002): 384–396, https://doi.org/10.1016/S0022-1031(02)00006-9; B. K. Payne, "Conceptualizing Control in Social Cognition: How Executive Functioning Modulates the Expression of Automatic Stereotyping." *Journal of Personality and Social Psychology* 89, no 4, (2005): 488.

14. L. E. Williams, J. A. Bargh, C. C. Nocera, and J. R. Gray, "The Unconscious Regulation of Emotion: Nonconscious Reappraisal Goals Modulate Emotional Reactivity," *Emotion* 9, no. 6 (2009): 847. For reviews of automatic strategy use, see I. B. Mauss, S. A. Bunge, and J. J. Gross, "Automatic Emotion Regulation," *Social and Personality Psychology Compass* 1, no. 1 (2007): 146–167, https://doi.org/10.1111/j.1751-9004.2007.00005.x; A. Gyurak, J. J. Gross, and A. Etkin, "Explicit and Implicit Emotion Regulation: A Dual-Process Framework," *Cognition and Emotion* 25, no. 3 (2011): 400–412, https://doi.org/10.1080/02699931.2010.544160.

15. See I. S. Gallo, A. Keil, K. C. McCulloch, B. Rockstroh, and P. M. Gollwitzer, "Strategic Automation of Emotion Regulation," *Journal of Personality and Social Psychology* 96, no. 1 (2009): 11.

16. See A. Etkin, T. Egner, D. M. Peraza, E. R. Kandel, and J. Hirsch, "Resolving Emotional Conflict: A Role for the Rostral Anterior Cingulate Cortex in Modulating Activity in the Amygdala," *Neuron* 51, no. 6 (2006): 871–882.

17. For a review of the literature on phantom limb pain, see B. Subedi and G. T. Grossberg, "Phantom Limb Pain: Mechanisms and Treatment Approaches," *Pain Research and Treatment* (2011): 864,605, https://doi.org/10.1155/2011/864605.

Chapter 9: Talking to Ourselves

1. S. S. Carson, C. E. Cox, S. Wallenstein, L. C. Hanson, M. Danis, J. A. Tulsky, E. Chai, and J. E. Nelson, "Effect of Palliative Care–Led Meetings for Families of Patients with Chronic Critical Illness: A Randomized Clinical Trial," *JAMA* 316, no. 1 (2016): 51–62.

2. H. G. Prigerson, M. Viola, C. R. Brewin, C. Cox, D. Ouyang, M. Rogers, C. X. Pan, et al., "Enhancing and Mobilizing the Potential for Wellness and Emotional Resilience (EMPOWER) Among Surrogate Decision-Makers of ICU Patients: Study Protocol for a Randomized Controlled Trial," *Trials* 20, no. 1 (2019): 408.

3. For the review of interventions attempting to increase optimism, see J. M. Malouff and N. S. Schutte, "Can Psychological Interventions Increase Optimism? A Meta-Analysis," *Journal of Positive Psychology* 12, no. 6 (2017): 594–604, https://doi.org/10.1080/17439760.2016.1221122. For the best-possible-self intervention, see Y. M. C. Meevissen, M. L. Peters, and H. J. E. M. Alberts, "Become More Optimistic by Imagining a Best Possible Self: Effects of a Two Week Intervention," *Journal of Behavior Therapy and Experimental Psychiatry* 42, no. 3 (2011): 371–378, https://doi.org/10.1016/j.jbtep.2011.02.012.

4. See N. Garnefski, V. Kraaij, M. Benoist, Z. Bout, E. Karels, and A. Smit, "Effect of a Cognitive Behavioral Self-Help Intervention on Depression, Anxiety, and Coping Self-Efficacy in People with Rheumatic Disease," *Arthritis Care and Research* 65, no. 7 (2013): 1077–1084; M. A. Martin, C. D. Catrambone, R. A. Kee, A. T. Evans, L. K. Sharp, C. Lyttle, C. Rucker-Whitaker, K. B. Weiss, J. J. Shannon, and the CHIRAH investigative team, "Improving Asthma Self-Efficacy: Developing and Testing a Pilot Community-Based Asthma Intervention for African American Adults," *Journal of Allergy and Clinical Immunology* 123, no. 1 (2009): 153–159.e3; C. Laureano, H. W. Grobbelaar, and A. W. Nienaber, "Facilitating the Confidence in Coping and Psychological Well-Being of Student Rugby Players," *South African Journal of Psychology* 44, no. 4 (2014): 483–497, https://doi.org/10.1016/j.jaci.2008.10.057; S. R. Liu and M. Kia-Keating, "Improving Confidence in Coping Among Distressed Students After Exposure to University Mass Violence: A Pilot Online Intervention," *Journal of College Student Psychotherapy* 32, no. 3 (2018): 199–219.

5. See M. Boekaerts, "The Adaptable Learning Process: Initiating and Maintaining Behavioural Change," *Applied Psychology* 41, no. 4 (1992): 377–397; M. Gregoire, "Is It a Challenge or a Threat? A Dual-Process Model of Teachers' Cognition and Appraisal Processes During Conceptual Change," *Educational Psychology Review* 15, no. 2 (2003): 147–179.

6. J. Tomaka, J. Blascovich, J. Kibler, and J. M. Ernst, "Cognitive and Physiological Antecedents of Threat and Challenge Appraisal," *Journal of Personality and Social Psychology* 73 (1997): 63–72.

7. See I. S. Gallo, A. Keil, K. C. McCulloch, B. Rockstroh, and P. M. Gollwitzer, "Strategic Automation of Emotion Regulation," *Journal of Personality and Social Psychology* 96, no. 1 (2009): 11; T. L. Webb and P. Sheeran, "How Do Implementation Intentions Promote Goal Attainment? A Test of Component Processes," *Journal of Experimental Social Psychology* 43, no. 2 (2007): 295–302, https://doi.org/10.1016/j.jesp.2006.02.001.

8. To capture the modulation of emotional feelings, we needed to include relatively objective measures, such as heart rate and facial electromyography. See

Z. Zhu and G. A. Bonanno, "Affective Flexibility: Relations to Expressive Flexibility, Feedback, and Depression," *Clinical Psychological Science* 5, no. 6 (2017), https://doi.org/10.1177/2167702617717337.

9. P. E. S. Schartau, T. Dalgleish, and B. D. Dunn, "Seeing the Bigger Picture: Training in Perspective Broadening Reduces Self-Reported Affect and Psychophysiological Response to Distressing Films and Autobiographical Memories," *Journal of Abnormal Psychology* 118, no. 1 (2009): 15.

10. S. Christou-Champi, T. F. D. Farrow, and T. L. Webb, "Automatic Control of Negative Emotions: Evidence That Structured Practice Increases the Efficiency of Emotion Regulation," *Cognition and Emotion* 29, no. 2 (2015): 319–331, https://doi.org/10.1080/02699931.2014.901213.

11. See E.-W. Park, F. Tudiver, J. K. Schultz, and T. Campbell, "Does Enhancing Partner Support and Interaction Improve Smoking Cessation? A Meta-Analysis," *Annals of Family Medicine* 2, no. 2 (2004): 170–174; N. El-Bassel, A. Ivanoff, R. F. Schilling, L. Gilbert, D. Borne, and D.-R. Chen, "Preventing HIV/AIDS in Drug-Abusing Incarcerated Women Through Skills Building and Social Support Enhancement: Preliminary Outcomes," *Social Work Research* 19, no. 3 (1995): 131–141.

12. B. H. O'Connell, D. O'Shea, and S. Gallagher, "Enhancing Social Relationships Through Positive Psychology Activities: A Randomised Controlled Trial," *Journal of Positive Psychology* 11, no. 2 (2016): 149–162.

13. For more on self-talk, see Alexander T. Latinjak, "Locating Self-Talk in the Knowledge Map of Sport and Exercise Psychology," in *Self-Talk in Sport*, ed. Alexander T. Latinjak and Antonis Hatzigeorgiadis, 1–10 (New York: Routledge, 2020); Julian Fritsch and Darko Jekauc, "Self-Talk and Emotion Regulation," in Latinjak and Hatzigeorgiadis, *Self-Talk in Sport*, 64–76; Ellen L. Usher and Dale H. Schunk, "Social Cognitive Theoretical Perspective of Self-Regulation," in *Handbook of Self-Regulation of Learning and Performance*, 2nd ed., ed. Dale H. Schunk and Jeffrey A. Greene, 19–35 (New York: Routledge, 2018).

14. I. Senay, D. Albarracín, and K. Noguchi, "Motivating Goal-Directed Behavior Through Introspective Self-Talk: The Role of the Interrogative Form of Simple Future Tense," *Psychological Science* 21, no. 4 (2010): 499–504, https://doi.org/10.1177/0956797610364751; P. K. Oleś, T. M. Brinthaupt, R. Dier, and D. Polak, "Types of Inner Dialogues and Functions of Self-Talk: Comparisons and Implications," *Frontiers in Psychology* 11 (2020): 227.

15. For a readable summary of self-talk, and, in particular, distanced self-talk, see Ethan Kross, *Chatter: The Voice in Our Head. Why It Matters, and How to Harness It* (New York: Crown, 2020). For more on the research on distanced self-talk, see E. Kross, E. Bruehlman-Senecal, J. Park, A. Burson, A. Dougherty, H. Shablack, R. Bremner, J. Moser, and O. Ayduk, "Self-Talk as a Regulatory Mechanism: How You Do It Matters," *Journal of Personality and Social Psychology* 106, no. 2 (2014): 304; A. Orvell, B. D. Vickers, B. Drake, P. Verduyn, O. Ayduk, J. Moser, J. Jonides, and E. Kross, "Does Distanced Self-Talk Facilitate Emotion Regulation Across a Range of Emotionally Intense Experiences?," *Clinical*

Psychological Science (2020), https://doi.org/10.1177/2167702620951539; A. Orvell, Ö. Ayduk, J. S. Moser, S. A. Gelman, and E. Kross, "Linguistic Shifts: A Relatively Effortless Route to Emotion Regulation?," *Current Directions in Psychological Science* 28, no. 6 (2019): 567–573.

16. James C. Coyne, Camille B. Wortman, and Darrin R. Lehman, "The Other Side of Support: Emotional Overinvolvement and Miscarried Helping," in *Marshaling Social Support: Formats, Processes, and Effects*, ed. Benjamin H. Gottlieb, 305–330 (Thousand Oaks, CA: Sage, 1988); J. C. Coyne, "Depression and the Response of Others," *Journal of Abnormal Psychology* 85 (1976): 186–193, https://doi.org/10.1037/0021-843X.85.2.186; E. D. Diminich and G. A. Bonanno, "Faces, Feelings, Words: Divergence Across Channels of Emotional Responding in Complicated Grief," *Journal of Abnormal Psychology* 123 (2014): 350–361.

Chapter 10: And Then There Was a Global Pandemic

1. "Report of the WHO-China Joint Mission on Coronavirus Disease 2019 (COVID-19)," February 16–24, 2020, www.who.int/docs/default-source/coronaviruse/who-china-joint-mission-on-covid-19-final-report.pdf. See also Derrick Bryson Taylor, "A Timeline of the Coronavirus," *New York Times*, January 10, 2021, www.nytimes.com/article/coronavirus-timeline.html.

2. "Cumulative Reported Cases of Probable SARS, 1 November 2002–11 July 2003," World Health Organization, www.who.int/csr/sars/country/2003_07_11/en.

3. K.-S. Yuen, Z.-W. Ye, S.-Y. Fung, C.-P. Chan, and D.-Y. Jin, "SARS-CoV-2 and COVID-19: The Most Important Research Questions," *Cell and Bioscience* 10, no. 40 (2020), https://doi.org/10.1186/s13578-020-00404-4.

4. R. Woelfel, V. M. Corman, W. Guggemos, M. Seilmaier, S. Zange, M. A. Müller, D. Niemeyer, et al., "Virological Assessment of Hospitalized Cases of Coronavirus Disease 2019," *MedRxiv*, 2020.03.05.20030502, https://doi.org/10.1101/2020.03.05.20030502.

5. B. Carey and J. Glanz, "Travel from New York City Seeded Wave of U.S. Outbreaks," *New York Times*, May 7, 2020, www.nytimes.com/2020/05/07/us/new-york-city-coronavirus-outbreak.html.

6. W. Wan, "The Coronavirus Pandemic Is Pushing America into a Mental Health Crisis," *Washington Post*, May 4, 2020, www.washingtonpost.com/health/2020/05/04/mental-health-coronavirus.

7. J. Aschenbach, "Coronavirus Is Harming the Mental Health of Tens of Millions of People in the U.S., New Poll Finds," *Washington Post*, April 2, 2020, www.washingtonpost.com/health/coronavirus-is-harming-the-mental-health-of-tens-of-millions-of-people-in-us-new-poll-finds/2020/04/02/565e6744-74ee-11ea-85cb-8670579b863d_story.html; A. Kirzinger, A. Kearney, L. Hamel, and M. Brodie, "KFF Health Tracking Poll—Early April 2020: The Impact of Coronavirus on Life in America," Kaiser Family Foundation (KFF), April 2, 2020, www.kff.org/coronavirus-covid-19/report/kff-health-tracking-poll-early-april-2020.

8. Aschenbach, "Coronavirus Is Harming the Mental Health of Tens of Millions."

9. These comments and others in this passage are quoted or paraphrased from a question-and-answer session I did that was published as an expert commentary on the website of the Association for Psychological Science: G. A. Bonanno, "APS Backgrounder Series. Psychological Science and COVID-19: Remaining Resilient During a Pandemic," Association for Psychological Science, March 30, 2020, www .psychologicalscience.org/news/backgrounders/backgrounder-1-resilient.html.

Index

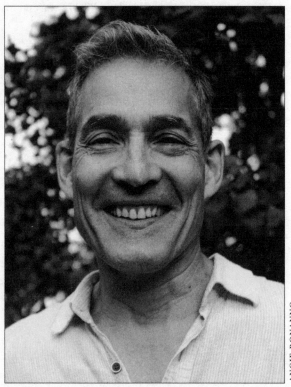

ANGIE BONANNO

GEORGE A. BONANNO is professor of clinical psychology, chair of the Department of Counseling and Clinical Psychology, and director of the Loss, Trauma, and Emotion Lab at Teachers College, Columbia University. He is the author of *The Other Side of Sadness: What the New Science of Bereavement Tells Us About Life After Loss* and lives in New York City.